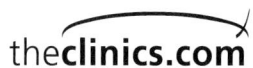

MEDICAL CLINICS OF NORTH AMERICA

Emergencies in the Outpatient Setting: Part I

GUEST EDITORS
Robert L. Rogers, MD
Joseph P. Martinez, MD

March 2006 • Volume 90 • Number 2

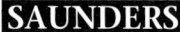

An Imprint of Elsevier, Inc.
PHILADELPHIA LONDON TORONTO MONTREAL SYDNEY TOKYO

W.B. SAUNDERS COMPANY
A Division of Elsevier Inc.

1600 John F. Kennedy Boulevard • Suite 1800 • Philadelphia, Pennsylvania 19103-2899

http://www.theclinics.com

MEDICAL CLINICS OF NORTH AMERICA   Volume 90, Number 2
March 2006   ISSN 0025-7125
Editor: Rachel Glover   ISBN 1-4160-3528-1

Copyright © 2006 Elsevier Inc. All rights reserved. No part of this publication may be reproduced or transmitted in any form or by any means, electronic or mechanical, including photocopy, recording, or any information retrieval system, without written permission from the publisher.

Single photocopies of single articles may be made for personal use as allowed by national copyright laws. Permission of the publisher and payment of a fee is required for all other photocopying, including multiple or systematic copying, copying for advertising or promotional purposes, resale, and all forms of document delivery. Special rates are available for educational institutions that wish to make photocopies for non-profit educational classroom use. Permissions may be sought directly from Elsevier's Rights Department in Philadelphia, PA, USA at Tel.: (+1) 215-239-3804; Fax: (+1) 215-239-3805; E-mail: healthpermissions@elsevier.com. Requests may also be completed on-line via the Elsevier homepage (http://www.elsevier.com/locate/permissions). In the USA, users may clear permissions and make payments through the Copyright Clearance Center, Inc., 222 Rosewood Drive, Danvers, MA 01923, USA; Tel.: (+1) 978-750-8400; Fax: (+1) 978-750-4744, and in the UK through the Copyright Licensing Agency Rapid Clearance Service (CLARCS), 90 Tottenham Court Road, London W1P 0LP, UK; Tel.: (+44) 171-436-5931; Fax: (+44) 171-436-3986. Other countries may have a local reprographic rights agency for payments.

The ideas and opinions expressed in *Medical Clinics of North America* do not necessarily reflect those of the Publisher. The Publisher does not assume any responsibility for any injury and/or damage to persons or property arising out of or related to any use of the material contained in this periodical. The reader is advised to check the appropriate medical literature and the product information currently provided by the manufacturer of each drug to be administered to verify the dosage, the method and duration of administration, or contraindications. It is the responsibility of the treating physician or other health care professional, relying on independent experience and knowledge of the patient, to determine drug dosages and the best treatment for the patient. Mention of any product in this issue should not be construed as endorsement by the contributors, editors, or the Publisher of the product or manufacturers' claims.

Medical Clinics of North America (ISSN 0025-7125) is published bimonthly by Elsevier. Corporate and editorial offices: 1600 John F. Kennedy Boulevard, Suite 1800, Philadelphia, PA 19103-2899. Accounting and circulation offices: 6277 Sea Harbor Drive, Orlando, FL 32887-4800. Periodicals postage paid at Orlando, FL 32862, and additional mailing offices. Subscription prices are USD 145 per year for US individuals, USD 260 per year for US institutions, USD 75 per year for US students, USD 185 per year for Canadian individuals, USD 330 per year for Canadian institutions, USD 210 per year for international individuals, USD 330 per year for international institutions and USD 110 per year for Canadian and foreign students/residents. To receive student/resident rate, orders must be accompanied by name of affiliated institution, date of term, and the *signature* of program/residency coordinator on institution letterhead. Orders will be billed at individual rate until proof of status is received. Foreign air speed delivery is included in all *Clinics* subscription prices. All prices are subject to change without notice. POSTMASTER: Send address changes to *Medical Clinics of North America*, W.B. Saunders Company, Periodicals Fulfillment, Orlando, FL 32887-4800. **Customer Service: 1-800-654-2452 (US). From outside of the USA, call (+1) 407-345-1000. E-mail: hhspcs@harcourt.com.**

Reprints. For copies of 100 or more, of articles in this publication, please contact the Commercial Reprints Department, Elsevier Inc., 360 Park Avenue South, New York, New York 10010-1710. Tel.: (+1) (212) 633-3813; Fax: (+1) (212) 462-1935; E-mail: reprints@elsevier.com.

Medical Clinics of North America is also published in Spanish by McGraw-Hill Interamericana Editores S. A., P.O. Box 5-237, 06500 Mexico, D.F., Mexico.

Medical Clinics of North America is covered in *Index Medicus, Current Contents, ASCA, Excerpta Medica, Science Citation Index,* and *ISI/BIOMED.*

Printed in the United States of America.

GOAL STATEMENT

The goal of *Medical Clinics of North America* is to keep practicing physicians up to date with current clinical practice by providing timely articles reviewing the state of the art in patient care.

ACCREDITATION

The *Medical Clinics of North America* is planned and implemented in accordance with the Essential Areas and Policies of the Accreditation Council for Continuing Medical Education (ACCME) through the joint sponsorship of the University of Virginia School of Medicine and Elsevier. The University of Virginia School of Medicine is accredited by the ACCME to provide continuing medical education for physicians.

The University of Virginia School of Medicine designates this educational activity for a maximum of 90 category 1 credits per year, 15 category 1 credits per issue, toward the AMA Physician's Recognition Award. Each physician should claim only those credits that he/she actually spent in the activity.

The American Medical Association has determined that physicians not licensed in the US who participate in this CME activity are eligible for AMA PRA category 1 credit.

Category 1 credit can be earned by reading the text material, taking the CME examination online at *http://www.theclinics.com/home/cme*, and completing the evaluation. After taking the test, you will be required to review any and all incorrect answers. Following completion of the test and evaluation, your credit will be awarded and you may print your certificate.

FACULTY DISCLOSURE/CONFLICT OF INTEREST

The University of Virginia School of Medicine, as an ACCME accredited provider, endorses and strives to comply with the Accreditation Council for Continuing Medical Education (ACCME) Standards of Commercial Support, Commonwealth of Virginia statutes, University of Virginia policies and procedures, and associated federal and private regulations and guidelines on the need for disclosure and monitoring of proprietary and financial interests that may affect the scientific integrity and balance of content delivered in continuing medical education activities under our auspices.

The University of Virginia School of Medicine requires that all CME activities accredited through this institution be developed independently and be scientifically rigorous, balanced and objective in the presentation/discussion of its content, theories and practices.

All authors/editors participating in an accredited CME activity are expected to disclose to the readers relevant financial relationships with commercial entities occurring within the past 12 months (such as grants or research support, employee, consultant, stock holder, member of speakers bureau, etc.). The University of Virginia School of Medicine will employ appropriate mechanisms to resolve potential conflicts of interest to maintain the standards of fair and balanced education to the reader. Questions about specific strategies can be directed to the Office of Continuing Medical Education, University of Virginia School of Medicine, Charlottesville, Virginia.

The authors/editors listed below have identified no professional or financial affiliations for themselves or their spouse/partner:
Robert A. Barish, MD, FACEP, FACP; Walter G. Belleza, MD; Nancy Chawla, MD; Rachel Glover, Acquisitions Editor; Suzanne Kalman, MD; Joseph P. Martinez, MD; Jerry Naradzay, MD, FACEP; Jonathan S. Olshaker, MD; Laura Pimentel, MD, MMM, CPE; and, Robert L. Rogers; MD, FAAEM, FACEP, FACP.

The authors/editors listed below identified the following professional or financial affiliations for themselves or their spouse/partner:
Jack Gladstein, MD is on the speakers' bureau for GlaxoSmithKline.

Disclosure of Discussion of non-FDA approved uses for pharmaceutical products and/or medical devices:
The University of Virginia School of Medicine, as an ACCME provider, requires that all faculty presenters identify and disclose any "off label" uses for pharmaceutical and medical device products. The University of Virginia School of Medicine recommends that each physician fully review all the available data on new products or procedures prior to instituting them with patients.

TO ENROLL

To enroll in the Medical Clinics of North America Continuing Medical Education program, call customer service at 1-800-654-2452 or visit us online at *http://www.theclinics.com/home/cme*. The CME program is available to subscribers for an additional fee of USD 205.

FORTHCOMING ISSUES

May 2006
Emergencies in the Outpatient Setting: Part II
Robert L. Rogers, MD, and
Joseph P. Martinez, MD, *Guest Editors*

July 2006
Nanomedicine
Chiming Wei, MD, PhD, *Guest Editor*

September 2006
The Complex Patient
Frits J. Huyse, MD, PhD, and
Friedrich Stiefel, MD, *Guest Editors*

RECENT ISSUES

January 2006
Allergy
Anthony Montanaro, MD, *Guest Editor*

November 2005
Medical Toxicology
Christopher P. Holstege, MD, and
Daniel E. Rusyniak, MD, *Guest Editors*

September 2005
Minority Health and Disparities-Related Issues: Part II
Eddie L. Greene, MD, and
Charles R. Thomas, Jr., MD, *Guest Editors*

THE CLINICS ARE NOW AVAILABLE ONLINE!

Access your subscription at:
http://www.theclinics.com

EMERGENCIES IN THE OUTPATIENT SETTING: PART I

GUEST EDITORS

ROBERT L. ROGERS, MD, FAAEM, FACEP, FACP, Assistant Professor (Surgery), Division of Emergency Medicine; Director, Undergraduate Medical Education; and Associate Residency Director, Emergency Medicine, University of Maryland School of Medicine, Baltimore, Maryland

JOSEPH P. MARTINEZ, MD, Assistant Professor (Surgery), Division of Emergency Medicine, University of Maryland School of Medicine; and Assistant Medical Director, Adult Emergency Department, University of Maryland Medical System, Baltimore, Maryland

CONTRIBUTORS

ROBERT A. BARISH, MD, FACP, FACEP, Vice Dean, Office of the Dean, University of Maryland School of Medicine, Baltimore, Maryland

WALTER G. BELLEZA, MD, Assistant Professor (Surgery), Division of Emergency Medicine, University of Maryland School of Medicine, Baltimore, Maryland

NANCY CHAWLA, MD, Resident, Department of Emergency Medicine, Boston University Medical Center, Boston, Massachusetts

JACK GLADSTEIN, MD, Associate Professor (Pediatrics and Neurology), Department of Pediatrics, University of Maryland School of Medicine, Baltimore, Maryland

SUZANNE KALMAN, MD, Chief Resident, Division of Emergency Medicine, University of Maryland School of Medicine, Baltimore, Maryland

JERRY NARADZAY, MD, FACEP, Medical Director, Emergency Services, Maria Parham Medical Center, Henderson, North Carolina

JONATHAN S. OLSHAKER, MD, Chairman, Department of Emergency Medicine, Boston University Medical Center; and Professor, Boston University School of Medicine, Boston, Massachusetts

LAURA PIMENTEL, MD, MMM, CPE, Assistant Professor, Division of Emergency Medicine, University of Maryland School of Medicine; and Chairman, Department of Emergency Medicine, Mercy Medical Center, Baltimore, Maryland

EMERGENCIES IN THE OUTPATIENT SETTING: PART I

CONTENTS

Preface ix
Robert L. Rogers and Joseph P. Martinez

Headache 275
Jack Gladstein

> This article hopes to put the medical practitioner at ease when he or she is handed a chart with a chief complaint of headache. Headache is a broad topic, with multiple causes ranging from the most benign to life threatening. Severe pain, nausea, vomiting, photophobia, or phonophobia may be the result of a purely medical cause, but the patient may have serious psychologic issues that can act as triggers. Usually both are involved because headache can affect a patient's home life, work environment, and social interactions. Although most headaches are not emergent, the discussion offers an approach to rapid diagnosis so that the true emergencies can be recognized and treated appropriately and expeditiously.

Diagnosis and Management of Dizziness and Vertigo 291
Nancy Chawla and Jonathan S. Olshaker

> This article reviews the diagnostic approach to the dizzy patient, with emphasis on the differentiation of clinical emergencies. A thorough history and physical examination are often diagnostic in evaluating these patients. Peripheral causes of vertigo arise from abnormalities in the vestibular end organs and are usually benign. Central vertigo, on the other hand, requires more aggressive workup and treatment. Other sources of dizziness without vertiginous symptoms are also reviewed.

Approach to Ophthalmologic Emergencies 305
Jerry Naradzay and Robert A. Barish

> This article presents evaluation and treatment approaches to ophthalmologic conditions that are likely to be encountered in a

primary care office. These conditions can be organized by diagnostic category, symptoms, and location of complaint. By using one or a combination of these categories, the practitioner can provide appropriate, timely, and effective ophthalmologic evaluation and treatment. Acute conditions are categorized according to urgency of intervention.

Otolaryngologic Emergencies in the Outpatient Setting 329
Walter G. Belleza and Suzanne Kalman

Most patients who present with ear, nose, and throat diseases have self-limited diseases and are treated successfully on an outpatient basis, without complications. However, because of their anatomic location, complications may compromise airway, neurologic, and cardiovascular structures. The relative rarity, for example, of deep-space infections and intracranial complications may have clinical presentations that are unfamiliar to the physician, which may result in the misdiagnosis and delayed treatment of a potentially life-threatening condition among the elderly, the immunocompromised, alcoholics, and immigrants, who are more likely to have atypical presentations and are the least likely to seek regular medical care. This article familiarizes the physician with those potentially life-threatening pathologic processes that may present initially in an outpatient setting.

Orthopedic Trauma: Office Management of Major Joint Injury 355
Laura Pimentel

Orthopedic injuries are common reasons for visits to primary care physicians. Careful history and physical examination with intelligent use of imaging technology will arrive at the correct diagnosis in most patients. Many conditions may be definitively managed by the office internist. Others may be initially stabilized and referred to orthopedic surgeons for definitive care. Nondisplaced fractures, tendon injuries, sprains, and overuse syndromes are entities within the purview of the primary care internist. This review covers commonly encountered traumatic conditions of the major joints. Familiarity and confidence with diagnosis and management of these conditions in the internal medicine office is optimal for the care of the adult patient.

Index 383

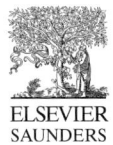

Preface
Emergencies in the Outpatient Setting: Part I

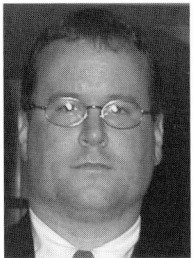 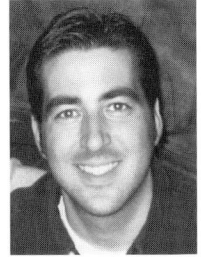

Robert L. Rogers, MD   Joseph P. Martinez, MD
Guest Editors

The evaluation of patients in the outpatient setting frequently results in the need to transport them to the emergency department (ED) for definitive diagnosis and management. Many chief complaints and specific disease entities are more easily managed in the ED due to the availability of airway and resuscitation equipment and access to specialty consultant care. Any discussion of emergent patient presentations would be remiss without discussing the obvious fact that many of the urgent and emergent conditions that develop in our patients are difficult to take care of in the office.

Primary care providers who see patients in the outpatient arena should be fully prepared to treat and stabilize ill patients to a higher level of care prior to transport. Furthermore, these providers must have concrete knowledge as to what conditions should be managed in the ED and what complaints and entities are best handled in the office to avoid unnecessary transport and ED overcrowding. Finally, there is a need for the primary care physician to be familiar with and understand subtle and atypical presentations of disease as well as the classic appearance. Although many patients will be quickly transported to the ED for stabilization, diagnosis, and admission, it is the outpatient physician's obligation to recognize whether a potential life threat exists in the first place.

The main goal of Part I of this double issue is to review some common urgent and emergent conditions that present to primary care offices. Topics of discussion include, (1) what conditions can and should be treated in the office without necessitating patient transport; (2) what entities require urgent or emergent transfer to the ED; (3) how to prepare your office for an emergency; and (4) what some of the "can't miss" entities could be that primary care physicians should be familiar with. With these in mind, Part I focuses on topics that are common and potentially life- or limb-threatening. Our goal is to provide a useful resource for the outpatient physician on what to do when faced with certain urgent and emergent patient complaints and presentations.

In the pages that follow, several common patient complaints and presentations will be discussed as they relate to how they are handled differently in the outpatient versus inpatient setting. The authors acknowledge that several of the articles included in this double issue cover topics that, on the surface, appear to be only appropriate for ED evaluation. For example, why were we compelled to discuss arrhythmias, pulmonary embolism, myocardial infarction, aortic dissection, spinal cord compression, or extremity fractures? Are any of these entities taken care of in the office setting? The answer is a resounding, "No." However, patients with these and numerous other conditions present initially to a primary care provider's office. Outpatient practitioners should be well aware that they are, to some degree, on the front line of patient care as much as emergency physicians, and are poised to make a tremendous difference in the lives of patients who seek medical attention for urgent and emergent problems. Prompt recognition of emergent medical and surgical conditions often starts with simply considering what potential diagnoses may be present and in what setting would be most appropriate for patient care. So, although many of these entities are dismissed from the office as quickly as they entered, it is important to note that the primary care physician can make a difference by being knowledgeable of the acute care issues at hand and working under the assumption that a limb- or life-threat is present until proven otherwise. We hope that Part I of this double issue proves useful in refreshing or providing that very knowledge.

Robert L. Rogers, MD
Assistant Professor (Surgery), Division of Emergency Medicine
Director, Undergraduate Medical Education
Associate Residency Director, Emergency Medicine
University of Maryland School of Medicine
Baltimore, MD, USA
E-mail address: rrogers@medicine.umaryland.edu

Joseph P. Martinez, MD
Assistant Professor (Surgery), Division of Emergency Medicine
University of Maryland School of Medicine

Assistant Medical Director, Adult Emergency Department
University of Maryland Medical System
Baltimore, MD, USA
E-mail address: jmartine@umaryland.edu

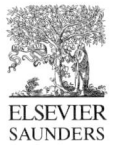

Headache

Jack Gladstein, MD*

Department of Pediatrics, University of Maryland School of Medicine, Baltimore, MD, USA

This article hopes to put the medical practitioner at ease when he or she is handed a chart with a chief complaint of headache. Headache is a broad topic, with multiple causes ranging from the most benign to life threatening. Severe pain, nausea, vomiting, photophobia, or phonophobia may be the result of a purely medical reason, but the patient may have serious psychologic issues that can act as triggers. Usually both medical and psychologic causes are involved because headache can affect the patient's home life, work environment, and social interactions. Although most forms of headache are not emergent, this discussion offers an approach to rapid diagnosis so that the true emergencies can be recognized and treated appropriately and expeditiously.

Diagnosis

All headache fits into four distinct patterns. Rothner's [1] model divides headache into acute, acute recurrent, chronic progressive, and chronic nonprogressive, as shown in Fig. 1 (time is measured in days on the x-axis, and headache severity is measured on an arbitrary scale on the y-axis). Because the acute recurrent pattern is seen most commonly in the office setting, that pattern is discussed first (Fig. 2).

Migraine

In the Landmark Study, patients who presented with a chief complaint of migraine had a final diagnosis of migraine [2]; patients whose chief complaint was sinus headache had a diagnosis of migraine; and patients whose chief complaint was tension-type headache left with a diagnosis of migraine.

---

* Department of Pediatrics, University of Maryland School of Medicine, 22 South Greene Street, Baltimore, MD 21201.
  E-mail address: jgladstein@som.umaryland.edu

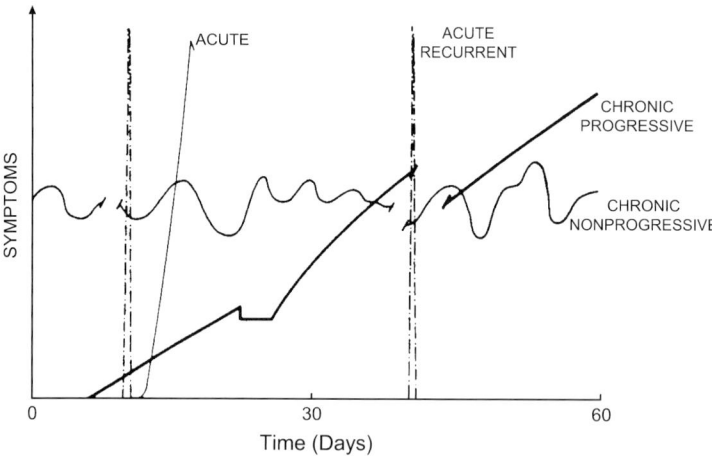

Fig. 1. All headache fits in one of these four categories. (*Adapted from* Rothner AD. Headaches in children and adolescents: update 2001. Semin Pediatr Neurol 2001;8:2–6; with permission.)

What this shows is that migraine is prevalent and underdiagnosed. In a population study by Lipton and colleagues [3], migraine is underdiagnosed by approximately 50% [1], yet the diagnosis is easy. The criteria include more than five episodes of headache lasting from 4 to 72 hours with nausea or vomiting, photophobia and phonophobia, and the inability to exercise strenuously; pain is typically unilateral but does not necessarily need to be. Symptoms that are even easier to diagnose as migraine are bad pain with autonomic symptoms, and supporting the diagnosis are a positive

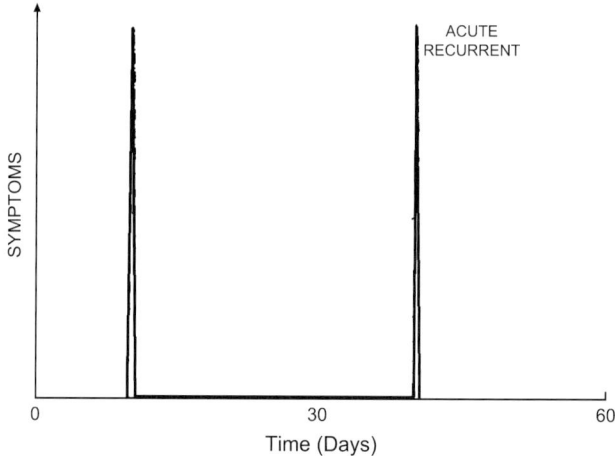

Fig. 2. Migraine and tension-type headache fit this pattern. (*Adapted from* Rothner AD. Headaches in children and adolescents: update 2001. Semin Pediatr Neurol 2001;8:2–6; with permission.)

family history and the need to rest. Note that location is not mentioned. Although classic teaching locates headaches as a unilateral frontal phenomenon, most headaches can be bilateral, temporal, occipital, or holocranial. When obtaining a family history, it is important to ask whether the affected family members had headache not migraine because other family members may have been misdiagnosed as well. To ascertain the degree of disability during an attack, ask the patient whether he or she could run up and down the stairs a few times during an episode. Migraine is a disease of young people, with a peak prevalence in the first few decades of life (Fig. 3). Migraine can occur with or without an aura, although most people have migraine without aura. Migraine aura, when present, is usually stereotypical. A migraine attack can begin with some warning. Patients may feel sluggish, hungry, or experience difficulty with finding words, which they will report in retrospect. There is a feeling of doom similar to that seen in seizure patients. An aura, however, is a memorable phenomenon. There are wavy lines that start peripherally and move across the visual field, usually sparing the midline. This was coined "fortification spectra," because forts were built with jagged outpouchings to protect a larger periphery. Headache usually begins 30 minutes or so after the onset of the visual aura. Migraine with aura is easily diagnosed, but most migraineurs do not experience this phenomenon. Migraine without aura is just as easy to diagnose if the paradigm "acute recurrent headache that stops what you are doing and has autonomic symptoms" is remembered. Other common autonomic symptoms include dizziness, lightheadedness, pallor, or purple bags around the eyes. If a patient brings a family member, the person should be asked whether he or she can tell just by looking that the patient has a headache.

There are rare cases of patients who have focal neurologic deficits when during their migraine episode. If a patient comes into the office with hemiplegia or ophthalmoplegia along with a severe headache, migraine is

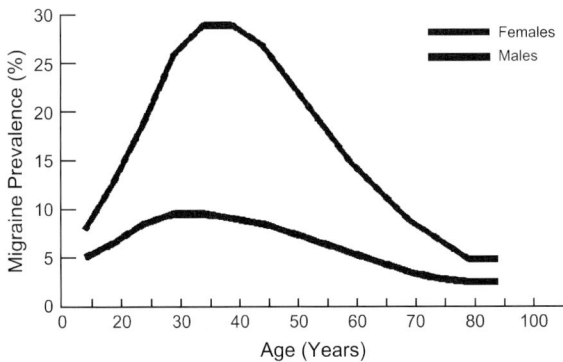

Fig. 3. The prevalence of migraine is an inverted U-shaped curve that peaks in middle life. Migraine is more prevalent in females (*top line*) than in males (*bottom line*) at all ages after puberty.

obviously a diagnosis of exclusion, whereas migraine with and without aura can be diagnosed confidently, without any tests. Patients who have such focal neurologic deficits need a work-up to exclude stroke, transient ischemic attack, or collagen vascular disease. Once these have been ruled out, however, complicated migraine exists in four forms. Hemiplegic migraine has an acute recurrent pattern with autonomic symptoms and hemiplegia. Ophthalmoplegic migraine has a recurrent pattern, autonomic symptoms, and double vision. On physical examination, extraocular movements are not intact. In basilar artery migraine, there are neurologic signs attributable to the distribution of the basilar system, so patients may be dizzy, lose consciousness, or be confused. A rare type of complicated migraine is referred to as "Alice in Wonderland" syndrome. In this condition, the patient complains of distortions of objects, and objects appear too big or too small. Some hypothesize that Lewis Carroll suffered from this condition.

In all forms of migraine, an assessment of the time of day is not that helpful. Some patients routinely wake in the middle of the night, some get worse as the day goes on, and some have no predictable pattern. Triggers vary from person to person. A long list of triggers has been implicated. The present author tells patients that, as a migraineurs, they are more susceptible to triggers. In effect, they have a sensitive autonomic system that responds to triggers with migraine. Headache sufferers need to eat, exercise, and sleep regularly. Some foods to avoid include caffeine, monosodium glutamate (MSG), chocolate, cheese, and sulfites. However, adhering to this diet is onerous. An elimination trial is a better option for most patients, in which one type of food is eliminated and then a judgment is made about whether there was a difference If not, the potentially migrainogenic food can be reintroduced in moderation. Migraineurs have a heightened sensitivity to flickering lights in the room, startle more easily, and have more sensitive skin interictally [4].

During a migraine attack, if left to oneself, a migraineur will need to retreat to a dark and quiet place in an attempt to decrease external stimulation. Patients will often want to lie down. In the past, treatment consisted of helping patients to sleep. Now, with the advent of triptan medication, patients should go back to work or school as part of their treatment plan.

Tension-type headache

In the acute recurrent pattern is the tension-type headache (TTH), which has no autonomic symptoms. Patients do not have nausea, vomiting, photophobia, or phonophobia and do not need to rest. The questions are, are tension and migraine two distinct entities or is tension just mild migraine? Both are exacerbated by stress, get worse as the day goes on, usually have no aura, and often respond to the same medications. This is not an academic question because, if we believe that tension is mild migraine, then migraine medications may be in order. To answer this question, Cady and colleagues

[5] analyzed a small group of protocol violators during a sumatriptan (Imitrex) trial. These subjects took their placebo or triptan when they were having a tension-type headache rather than the migraine, as the trial dictated. The authors found that the tension-type headache patients responded significantly better to triptan than placebo. The study concluded that most patients who have primary headache exist on a spectrum, in which the onset of headaches is either migraine or the tension-type, but very few patients have either pure migraine or pure tension-type headaches; this is now called the spectrum study [5].

Chronic nonprogressive headache

Rothner's [1] second category of headaches is called nonprogressive headaches. In this pattern, a patient has 15 days per month of at least 4 hours of headache per day. This pattern is often referred to as chronic daily headache (CDH) (Fig. 4). Silberstein and colleagues [6] divided this pattern into four categories. In transformed or chronic migraine, there is usually a long period of transformation to a chronic condition. There are still days of migraine with autonomic symptoms. The pearl here is that these migraine-like episodes still respond to migraine-specific medications. In children, the period of transformation from first migraine to CDH is, on average, 2 years, whereas in adults, the period of transformation is, on average, 10 years [7]. In chronic tension-type headache, there is a history of pure tension-type headache and then a transformation to a daily or near daily pattern. There was never and there are never any autonomic symptoms.

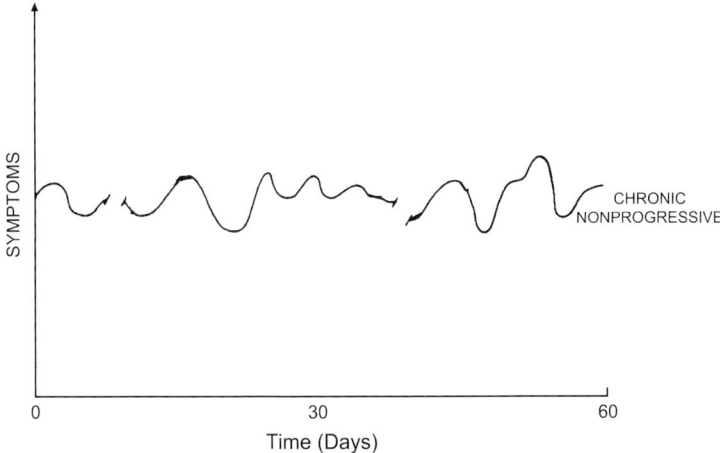

Fig. 4. Chronic daily headache fits this pattern. There may or may not be acute migraine attacks interspersed. (*Adapted from* Rothner AD. Headaches in children and adolescents: update 2001. Semin Pediatr Neurol 2001;8:2–6; with permission.)

In persistent daily headache, as opposed to the first two types, there is no history of acute recurrent headache. There is often a preceding viral infection or trauma and then a mysterious onset of daily headache. This is a difficult problem that is often refractory to standard treatment, even in the most capable of hands [8]. A fourth and very rare form of CDH is hemicrania continua, in which headache pain happens for short bursts daily, is responsive to indomethacin, and is always unilateral.

Common to all four of these categories of the CDH pattern is the absence of a positive work-up, and the possibility that the condition was exacerbated by medication overuse. The issues of prevalent medication overuse in CDH patients and the role of medication are in debate. Warner [9] believes that all chronic headaches can be stopped with medication washout and that medication overuse is the cause of the chronicity. Other authors believe that this is true for a small segment of the patients and that the use of chronic pain medicine is the inevitable consequence of having chronic pain; it is a symptom rather than a cause. Either way, removal of chronic pain medications should be an integral part of treatment for those patients who have chronic headache.

Acute headache

When someone presents with a new onset of headache for the first time, it is important to make sure that the patient is not in the early stages of a life-threatening illness. Reassuringly, most patients in this category are easily diagnosed (Fig. 5). The most common reason a patient who has a headache reports to an emergency department is viral syndrome, so the presence of fever and headache in an examination with otherwise normal findings is

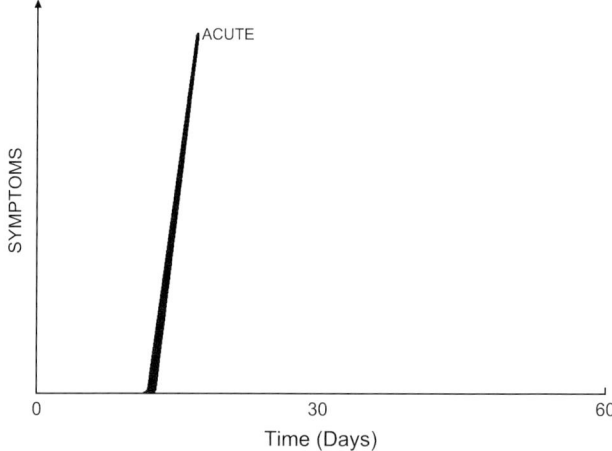

Fig. 5. Acute headache may be serious or benign in nature. (*Adapted from* Rothner AD. Headaches in children and adolescents: update 2001. Semin Pediatr Neurol 2001;8:2–6; with permission.)

not too worrisome. Similarly, if someone has a fever and stiff neck in the summer, it is most probably viral meningitis. If someone has fever and a change in mental status, they need to be worked up for encephalitis.

How to save someone's life

Rapidly diagnosing subarachnoid hemorrhage is heroic, whereas missing the diagnosis is often tragic. Luckily, when a patient presents with the sentinel bleed that precedes the rupture of an aneurysm, the scripted complaint is that they have the worst headache of their life. They will also say that the pain came on within seconds. Whereas a migraine builds for over an hour, this headache came immediately to full force. This "thunderclap headache" can be accompanied by a low-grade fever and stiff neck because blood in the subarachnoid space can act as a local irritant and endogenous pyrogen. If the diagnosis is suspected, the patient needs an emergent CT scan and lumbar puncture (LP), with rapid neurosurgical consultation [10,11].

Other emergencies for acute headache include glaucoma and cavernous venous thrombosis [12]. In glaucoma, there is eye pain and a change in vision; in cavernous venous thrombosis, there is usually a history of ear-nose-throat surgery, localized nasal infection, or the use of medications that could cause a hypercoagulable state [13].

Chronic progressive headache

In the chronic progressive headache, pain has increased slowly and steadily over the course of weeks to months. This is the ominous headache of space-occupying lesions. As intracranial pressure (ICP) rises, it tends to become deregulated. Patients can tolerate only a very narrow range of ICP. Once the range is exceeded, pain increases. Coughing, straining in the bathroom, sneezing, or just bending forward may exacerbate the pain. Pain is often worse in the morning and then gets a little better as the day goes on. In this situation gravity is a friend. When a patient with a mass is recumbent all night, pressure creeps upward just enough to make the patient symptomatic. If a history of this pattern emerges, the work-up will include MRI, rather than CT, because MRI provides a better look at the posterior fossa. The differential of space-occupying lesions is beyond the scope of this article; however, a few pearls are in order: If there is a progressive loss of visual acuity, consider midline lesions, such as like craniopharyngioma, compressing the optic discs. If there is secondary amenorrhea, consider pituitary lesions. If there are café-au-lait spots, consider neurofibromatosis and its complications as a possibility. Primary intracranial hypertension, also known as pseudotumor cerebri, presents with this same pattern. If the clinician is not skilled at fundoscopy, observing spontaneous venous pulsations should reassure the examiner that the pressure is not too elevated. A patient who has the progressive pattern along with abnormal discs merits an LP with opening pressure (Fig. 6).

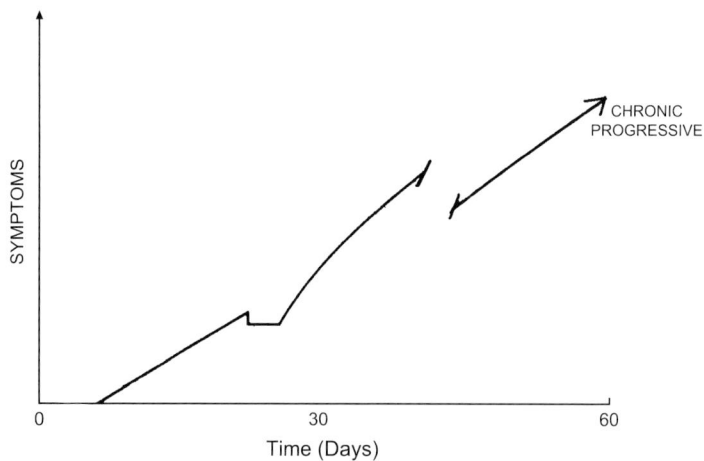

Fig. 6. Chronic progressive headache is usually ominous. (*Adapted from* Rothner AD. Headaches in children and adolescents: update 2001. Semin Pediatr Neurol 2001;8:2–6; with permission.)

Approach to the patient

With Rothner's [1] model in mind, the diagnosis should just take a few moments of office time. Having found the pattern, the differential diagnosis is quite manageable. One can then focus on disability. How have the headaches affected the patient and her family? Objective measures include the number of days of work or school missed, but other markers of disability include family function, curtailment of enjoyable activities, and a general description of what happens at home when the patient gets a headache. The Migraine Disability Assessment Questionnaire scale or the Headache Impact Test score can generate a disability score that can be followed over time [14].

Physical examination reassures both the clinician and patient while ensuring that nothing important is missed. Patients should be undressed and examined in a gown with underwear off because a careful inspection for café-au-lait spots and scoliosis may hint at intracranial pathology. Vital signs will help discover patients who have hypertension as well as Cushing's triad. The rest of the physical examination is standard. A thorough neurologic examination is indicated. Luckily, there are few surprises. If a history consistent with migraine is presented and the examination is normal, there is no need for further work-up [15]. Again, a worrisome history and an abnormal examination will lead to immediate work-up. The approach can be summarized with the acronym SNOOP (*s*ystemic symptoms, *n*eurological signs, *o*lder patient at onset [if older than 50 years, new migraine is uncommon], *o*nset is abrupt, *p*rior headache history is different). If SNOOPing results are negative, a patient has a primary headache and needs no further work-up. If a worrisome sign or symptom is elicited, further work-up is indicated.

Diagnostic pitfalls

Sinus versus migraine

Because the second branch of the trigeminal nerve innervates the nose, eyes, and maxillary sinus areas, a migraine can sometimes cause lacrimation, rhinorrhea, and sinus tenderness. If there are autonomic symptoms and the pattern is acute and recurrent, it is migraine not sinus disease. Sinus disease presents as fever, cough, and halitosis; it does not remit and return as migraine does [16].

Chiari malformation

As many as 10% of normal patients are shown to have Chiari malformation on MRI, so 10% of migraineurs would also have this diagnosis radiologically. This is an argument against scanning all headache patients. Symptomatic Chiari requiring neurosurgical intervention involves tingling of hands and feet during headache or headache that is consistently posterior in location [17].

Treatment

Once they are diagnosed, most patients will have migraine. The Landmark Study [2] shows that whether a chief complaint is migraine, tension, or sinus, the end diagnosis is migraine. Patients who have the pure tension-type headache do not seek medical help because these minor headaches can be treated easily and effectively with over-the-counter (OTC) medicines. Discussion therefore focuses on the treatment of migraine, which can be divided into acute, preventative, and general.

Acute migraine treatment

To understand acute treatment, a short review of pathophysiology will help [18]. Migraine is a race against the clock. The longer one waits, the less likely drugs will work [19]. In patients who are genetically susceptible, a trigger happens. This trigger begins a cascade, culminating in release of "inflammatory soup" from the trigeminovascular system. This soup inflames the meninges, (causing throbbing), tickles the salivatory nucleus, causing activation of the parasympathetic system, and eventually sends signals up to the trigeminal nucleus and then up to the cortex. This signal is mediated through the 5-hydroxytryptamine $(HT)_{1D}$ and $5HT_{1B}$ receptors. The depletion of serotonin caused by this trigger opens the gate of the receptor, causing the inflammation. Triptans are designer serotonin compounds that fool the receptor and shut it off, thereby stopping the release of the soup. This pathophysiology helps to explain why early treatment is so important: the more soup, the more inflammation. Up to this point, there is little recruitment of central processes. As a headache progresses, the trigeminal nucleus caudalis can fire independently. This is manifested in cutaneous allodynia. A patient will say that her hair hurts or that she cannot keep her glasses on or her coat on her shoulders. This is the phenotypic manifestation of a migraine evolving from a peripheral problem to a central one. Triptans do not work as well once central sensitization occurs [20].

With this pathophysiology as a backdrop, we can understand how migraine can best be treated. OTC drugs, such as ibuprofen, acetaminophen, and naproxen sodium do have a role. They are generally prostaglandin inhibitors and mitigate inflammation. They have their role early in a headache, while the stomach is still working properly. Once nausea is present, their efficacy dwindles. The pearl is to use higher doses of these drugs, assuming some gastroparesis has already taken place.

Before the availability of triptan drugs, combination drugs were prescribed in an attempt to put the migraineurs to bed and sleep off the headache. Drugs such as acetaminophen/isometheptene/dichloralphenazone and butalbital/acetaminophen/caffeine have gone out of favor because of their sedative effect and potential for overuse [21,22].

Headache treatment changed dramatically in 1993 with the introduction of the triptan drugs. Migraines could be treated with drugs that attacked the physiology directly and could get patients back to work and school quickly. The first triptan, sumatriptan (Imitrex) came out as subcutaneous injectable. It was followed by a nasal spray and tablet form. Other drugs soon followed. There are now seven triptans. Sumatriptan is available in a pill, nasal spray, and injection; zolmitriptan is available in nasal spray, melting tablet, and a conventional tablet; and rizatriptan is available in melting and conventional tablets. Almotriptan and eletriptan are available only as tablets. Naratriptan and frovatriptan are long-acting triptans that have a role in short-term prophylaxis (eg, menstrual migraine) or for patients who have relief with conventional triptan but then have a rapid recurrence. The choice of triptan is based on a combination of factors. Generally, injections and nasal sprays work faster and bypass the gut, whereas pills and melting tablets require the cooperation of the gastrointestinal (GI) tract. Also, generally, shots and nasal sprays may have more side effects, but their actions are more reliable and repeatable, whereas the variability of absorption through the GI tract makes these routes troublesome for some patients. In the United States, 80% of the triptan sold are pills. Reluctance to use parenteral forms continues to dominate the United States market (Table 1).

As stated earlier, teaching points for the migraine patient must stress the earliest use of headache medicine in an attack to prevent central sensitization. Treating headache early is the best prognosticator of success. Patients need to have permission to go right to a triptan if their headache is bad. Using an OTC pain reliever works for some patients, but their use delays good care for many others. Once the race is lost, triptan efficacy drops dramatically.

What to do when a patient says
  1. "My triptan did not work." ***Possible response:*** Perhaps you waited too long; perhaps you should increase the dose; or try a nasal inhaler or injection.

Table 1
Triptan formulations currently available

Triptan[a]	Tablet (mg)	Melt (mg)	Nasal (mg)	Subcutaneous (mg)
Almotriptan	6.25, 12.5	—	—	—
Eletriptan	20, 40	—	—	—
Frovatriptan	2.5	—	—	—
Naratriptan	1, 2.5	—	—	—
Rizatriptan	5, 10	5, 10	—	—
Sumatriptan	25, 50, 100	—	5, 20	6
Zolmitriptan	2.5, 5	2.5, 5	5	—

[a] Frovatriptan and naratriptan have longer half-lives and may be used for menstrual migraine prophylaxis, or for recurrence. Other drugs are shorter acting, to be used acutely only.

2. "My triptan worked but then the headache came right back with a vengeance." **Possible response:** Did you wait too long? You might want to try a long-acting triptan.
3. "My triptan worked the first time but not the second, and then it worked for the third attack but not the fourth." **Possible response:** Did you wait too long? Try a nasal spray or shot.
4. "Too many adverse events have occurred." **Possible response:** Try naratriptan or lower the dose of the triptan used presently.

Triptophobia

Triptophobia, or the irrational fear of using triptans, is caused by a number of factors. Side effects may frighten the patient. Chest symptoms, such as chest pain, and arm and jaw pain mimic the worrisome signs of an impending heart attack. Studies have examined patients who had these symptoms using electrocardiograms, Holter monitors, cardiac enzymes, and transesophageal echocardiography and found the results to be normal [23]. Doctors may be afraid of inducing harm in an otherwise healthy person. Unmasking cardiac disease with use of these drugs does not occur. The drugs are contraindicated in patients who are known to have coronary artery disease because there is a slight narrowing that occurs. In patients who have a high risk of coronary artery disease, a work-up must take place before prescribing triptans [24]. Otherwise, this is a disease of healthy young people, so for most patients these drugs offer no problems.

Because most migraineurs are women of childbearing age, pregnancy can happen for patients who take the drugs. There is a registry for patients to sign up should this happen. The drugs are not to be used currently during pregnancy because the registry has not yet enrolled enough patients to show that the drugs are safe. There have been no reported problems so far, however [25]. For the nursing mother, the drugs can be used with caution [26].

Migraine prevention strategies

Some people believe that anyone can get a migraine, if provoked. Migraineurs have a lower threshold than nonmigraineurs. Potential triggers to avoid include hunger, stress, change in sleep patterns, and certain foods containing sulfites and MSG. Migraineurs are therefore encouraged to eat and sleep regularly and avoid foods that may trigger their headaches. Stress reduction, good eating habits, and smoking cessation are encouraged for all patients (regardless of migraine status) [27].

The decision to use prophylactic drugs for a migraineur should be based on the severity and frequency of attacks after prescribing a triptan. Days of missed work or school in an average month are an easy measure to follow. Because a successful outcome of prophylactic treatment is considered to be a 50% drop in the frequency of headaches, the drugs we use for this purpose are not that good [28]. Picking the drug then should be based on what else is wrong with the patient. This comorbidity can help to choose some drugs and avoid others. For example, β-blockers exacerbate depression, asthma, and exercise intolerance. They should not be used for patients who have depression, the asthmatic patient, or an athlete [29]. Topiramate is a good choice for an obese person, whereas cyproheptadine or a tricyclic antidepressant would help a patient to gain weight [30–32]. Valproate, gabapentin, and topiramate are anticonvulsants, so they could help a patient with migraine and epilepsy [33]. Valproate is helpful in conduct disorder, so it could help a person with violence tendencies [34]. Newer antidepressants such as venlafaxine may help alleviate anxiety as well as depression [35].

Nonprescription medicines have been used as well. Feverfew, magnesium, coenzyme Q-10, and riboflavin may have a role in migraine prophylaxis [36]. Biofeedback relaxation, hypnosis, and cognitive therapy work well for patients who are motivated to practice on a daily basis [37]. In the present author's experience, busy, organized people like to take control of their lives and do well with these modalities, whereas people who tend to be disorganized and poor time managers cannot commit to the rigors of daily practice.

Treatment of tension-type headache

Patients who never get autonomic symptoms with their headache do not have migraine and will not respond to triptans. Patients who have migraines but experience a milder version without autonomic symptoms do respond to triptans. Basically, for this group, TTH is mild migraine. Because OTC drugs work well for mild headache, patients who have pure tension-type headaches seldom present in doctors' offices. Therefore, this diagnosis made in a physician's office is overrated. We can be fooled if headache occurs in the neck. If there are autonomic symptoms, it is still migraine, and a triptan should be prescribed [16].

Treatment of chronic daily headache

The first decision point for handling this problem is whether there is medication overuse [6]. The offending agent must be eliminated to achieve success. This can be done first or at the same time that a prevention drug or alternative therapy is initiated [38]. If a patient has chronic migraines, the bad headaches with autonomic symptoms must be treated like migraine, using migraine-selective drugs [39]. If a patient has chronic tension-type headaches, the migraine drugs will probably not work [40]. Again, the physician should pick a preventive regimen that gives treatment of other conditions and avoid drugs that may exacerbate underlying comorbidities. Stress management, psychotherapy, and other modalities may help as well. Many of these patients need referral to a headache clinic.

Treatment of status migranosus

Occasionally, a known migraineur will be unresponsive to standard treatment. This condition has been termed status migranosus. In this situation, options include intravenous (IV) fluids, dihydroergotamine combined with metoclopramide, IV valproate, IV magnesium, and corticosteroids [41–45]. When all else fails, a narcotic can be used with caution [46]. If the headache has broken, some patients may benefit from a long-term triptan prescription for 3 to 5 days to keep the headache from recurring [47].

Frequently asked questions in the office management of headache

Who needs a referral to a headache specialist?

There is no literature to address this question, so this is common sense advice for the practitioner. Referral is indicated when the diagnosis is unclear, the patient is not responding to the treatment at the practitioner's comfort level, the patient has CDH caused by medication overuse, or the patient has serious comorbidity.

What about cluster headache?

Cluster is easy to distinguish from migraine. Whereas the migraine patient retires to bed in the dark, a cluster patient is agitated. Cluster headache is unilateral, with lacrimation and rhinorrhea on the side of the pain [48].

What about pregnancy?

One third of migraine patients get better, one-third gets worse, and one third stays the same. Treatments are limited. Nonpharmacologic interventions are helpful, such as biofeedback, hypnosis, relaxation. Triptans have not yet been studied sufficiently to determine a safety rating. There is a triptan registry for patients to be followed who have been exposed to triptan before pregnancy was discovered. OTC drugs and opioids have been used safely. For prophylaxis, amitriptyline is safe until the third trimester [49].

What about menopause?

Headaches are often exacerbated in perimenopause, during which exaggerated swings of estrogen levels are the rule. The use of estrogen supplements will help the headaches, but such supplements should be used in conjunction with an internist or primary care physician who can explain the risks and benefits [50,51].

Who needs a CT scan?

A regular migraine patient does not need to undergo CT [15]. Patients who need to be scanned include those whose history or physical examination is suspicious, a patient who is older at the age of onset, or for a patient of any age if there is a change in headache pattern.

Summary

The patient who presents with headache can be diagnosed quickly and efficiently once the correct pattern has been identified. Most patients will have migraine, and treatment is based on the severity and disability. If the identified patient has significant disability, a medication that treats comorbidity should be prescribed. Patients who have a serious underlying disorder can be recognized by a thoughtful history and careful examination and can be worked up accordingly. Patients who have an acute new onset headache problem that requires immediate attention can be triaged and treated once their pattern and history are clear. Hopefully, increasing comfort levels with diagnosing headaches will allow the primary care practitioner to treat headache patients more effectively and efficiently.

References

[1] Rothner AD. Headaches in children and adolescents: update 2001. Semin Pediatr Neurol 2001;8:2–6.
[2] Tepper SJ, Dahlof CG, Dowson A, et al. Prevalence and diagnosis of migraine in patients consulting their physician with a complaint of headache: data from the Landmark Study. Headache 2004;44(9):856–64.
[3] Lipton RB, Stewart WF, Simon D. Medical consultation for migraine: results from the American Migraine Study. Headache 1998;38:87–96.
[4] Welch KMA, D'Andrea G, Tepley N, et al. The concept of migraine as a state of central neuronal hyperexcitability. Headache 1990;8:817–28.
[5] Cady RK, Lipton RB, Hall C, et al. Treatment of mild headache in disabled migraine sufferers: results of the Spectrum Study. Headache 2000;40(10):792–7.
[6] Silberstein SD, Lipton RB, Sliwinski M. Classification of daily and near-daily headaches: field trial of revised IHS criteria. Neurology 1996;47:871–5.

[7] Gladstein J, Holden EW. Chronic daily headache in children and adolescents: a 2 year prospective study. Headache 1996;36(6):349–51.
[8] Hershey AD, Powers SW, Bentti AL, et al. Characterization of chronic daily headaches in children in a multidisciplinary headache center. Neurology 2001;56(8):1032–7.
[9] Warner JS. The outcome of treating patients with suspected rebound headache. Headache 2001;41(7):685–92.
[10] Van Gijn J, Van Dongen KJ. The time course of aneurismal hemorrhage on computed tomograms. Neuroradiology 1982;23:153–6.
[11] Vermulen M, Hasan D, Blijenberg BG, et al. Xanthochromia after subarachnoid hemorrhage needs no revisitation. J Neurol Neurosurg Psychiatry 1989;52:826–8.
[12] Weinreb RN, Khaw PT. Primary open-angle glaucoma. Lancet 2004;363(9422):1711–20.
[13] de Brujin SF, Stam J, Vanderbroucke JP, for the Cerebral Venous Sinus Thrombosis Study Group Increased risk of cerebral venous sinus thrombosis with third-generation oral contraceptives. Lancet 1996;348:1623–5.
[14] Lipton RB, Bigal ME, Amatniek JC, et al. Tools for diagnosing migraine and measuring its severity. Headache 2004;44(5):387–98.
[15] Report of the Quality Standards Subcommittee of the American Academy of Neurology. Practice parameter: the utility of neuroimaging in the evaluation of headache in patients with normal neurological examinations. Neurology 1994;44:1353–4.
[16] Kaniecki RG. Migraine and tension-type headache: an assessment of challenges in diagnosis. Neurology 2002;58(9)(Suppl 6):S15–20.
[17] Milhorat TH, Chou MW, Trinidad EM, et al. Chiari I malformation redefined: clinical and radiographic findings for 364 symptomatic patients. Neurosurgery 1999;44(5):1005–17.
[18] Waeber C, Moskowitz MA. Therapeutic implications of central and peripheral neurologic mechanisms in migraine. Neurology 2003;61(8)(Suppl 4):S9–20.
[19] Burstein R, Collins B, Jakubowski M. Defeating migraine pain with triptans: a race against the development of cutaneous allodynia. Ann Neurol 2004;55(1):19–26.
[20] Burstein R. Deconstructing migraine headache into peripheral and central sensitization. Pain 2001;89(2–3):107–10.
[21] Wenzel RG, Sarvis CA. Do butalbital-containing products have a role in the management of migraine? Pharmacotherapy 2002;22(8):1029–35.
[22] Rapaport AM. Analgesic rebound headache. Headache 1988;28:662–5.
[23] Dodick DW, Martin VT, Smith T, et al. Cardiovascular tolerability and safety of triptans: a review of clinical data. Headache 2004;44(Suppl 1):S20–30.
[24] Papademetriou P. Cardiovascular risk and triptans. Headache 2004;44(Suppl 1):S31–9.
[25] Loder E. Safety of sumatriptan in pregnancy: a review of the data so far. CNS Drugs 2003; 17(1):1–7.
[26] Evans RW, Lipton RB. Topics in migraine management: a survey of headache specialists highlights some controversies. Neurol Clin 2001;19(1):1–21.
[27] Martin VT, Behbehani MM. Toward a rational understanding of migraine trigger factors. Med Clin North Am 2001;85(4):911–41.
[28] Bigal ME, Krymchantowski AV, Rapoport AM. New developments in migraine prophylaxis. Expert Opin Pharmacother 2003;4(4):433–43.
[29] Linde K, Rossnagel K. Propranolol for migraine prophylaxis. Cochrane Database Syst Rev 2004;2:CD003225.
[30] Swanson JW. Topiramate for migraine prevention. Curr Neurol Neurosci Rep 2005;5(2):77–8.
[31] Comer SD, Haney M, Fischman MW, et al. Cyproheptadine produced modest increases in total caloric intake by humans. Physiol Behav 1997;62(4):831–9.
[32] Colombo B, Annovazzi PO, Comi G. Therapy of primary headaches: the role of antidepressants. Neurol Sci 2004;25(Suppl 3):S171–5.
[33] Chronicle E, Mulleners W. Anticonvulsant drugs for migraine prophylaxis. Cochrane Database Syst Rev 2004;3:CD003226.

[34] Fava M. Psychopharmacologic treatment of pathologic aggression. Psychiatr Clin North Am 1997;20(2):427–51.
[35] Adelman LC, Adelman JU, Von Seggern R, et al. Venlafaxine extended release (XR) for the prophylaxis of migraine and tension-type headache: a retrospective study in a clinical setting. Headache 2000;40(7):572–80.
[36] Bianchi A, Salomone S, Caraci F, et al. Role of magnesium, coenzyme Q10, riboflavin, and vitamin B12 in migraine prophylaxis. Vitam Horm 2004;69:297–312.
[37] Penzien DB, Rains JC, Andrasik F. Behavioral management of recurrent headache: three decades of experience and empiricism. Appl Psychophysiol Biofeedback 2002;27(2):163–81.
[38] Young WB. Drug-induced headache. Neurol Clin 2004;22(1):173–84.
[39] Bussone G. Chronic migraine and chronic tension-type headache: different aspects of the chronic daily headache spectrum: clinical and pathogenetic considerations. Neurol Sci 2003;24(Suppl 2):S90–3.
[40] Goadsby P. Chronic tension-type headache. Clinical Evidence 2002;7:1145–52.
[41] Agostoni E, Santoro P, Frigerio R, et al. Management of headache in emergency room. Neurol Sci 2004;25(Suppl 3):S187–9.
[42] Callaham M, Raskin N. A controlled study of dihydroergotamine in the treatment of acute migraine headache. Headache 1986;26(4):168–71.
[43] Norton J. Use of intravenous valproate sodium in status migraine. Headache 2000;40(9): 755–7.
[44] Cete Y, Dora B, Ertan C, et al. A randomized prospective placebo-controlled study of intravenous magnesium sulphate vs. metoclopramide in the management of acute migraine attacks in the Emergency Department. Cephalalgia 2005;25(3):199–204.
[45] Monzillo PH, Nemoto PH, Costa AR, et al. Acute treatment of migraine in emergency room: comparative study between dexamethasone and haloperidol: preliminary results. Arq Neuropsiquiatr 2004;62(2B):513–8.
[46] Ziegler DK. Opioids in headache treatment: is there a role? Neurol Clin 1997;15(1):199–207.
[47] Gobel H, Winter P, Boswell D, et al. for the Naratriptan International Recurrence Study Group. Comparison of naratriptan and sumatriptan in recurrence-prone migraine patients. Clin Ther 2000;22(8):981–9.
[48] Rozen TD. Cluster headache: diagnosis and treatment. Curr Neurol Neurosci Rep 2005;5(2): 99–104.
[49] Martin SR, Foley MR. Approach to the pregnant patient with headache. Clin Obstet Gynecol 2005;48(1):2–11.
[50] Misakian AL, Langer RD, Bensenor IM, et al. Postmenopausal hormone therapy and migraine headache. J Womens Health 2003;12(10):1027–36.
[51] Silberstein SD. Headache and female hormones: what you need to know. Curr Opin Neurol 2001;14(3):323–33.

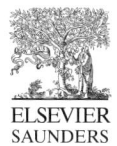

Diagnosis and Management of Dizziness and Vertigo

Nancy Chawla, MD[a],*, Jonathan S. Olshaker, MD[a,b]

[a]*Department of Emergency Medicine, Boston University Medical Center, Boston, MA, USA*
[b]*Boston University School of Medicine, Boston, MS, USA*

Dizziness is the third most common complaint among all outpatients and the single most common complaint among patients older than 75 years [1]. These patients present to psychiatry clinics, emergency departments, and outpatient offices. In all of these settings, the amount of time that the clinician has to spend with the patient is limited. Chronic cases average five physician visits without resolution (Charles Yanofsky, MD, unpublished data, 2004). For the patient, the ongoing dizziness and imbalance can lead to loss of function, falls, and injuries.

The evaluation of the dizzy patient can certainly be overwhelming for any clinician. Few other complaints have such a broad differential. Dizziness as a chief complaint encompasses weakness, presyncope, neurologic impairment, vertigo, visual disturbance, and psychologic illness. Often difficult and time-consuming to handle, the dizzy patient is commonly referred to medical specialists. Although otolaryngology, neurology, and cardiology all play an important role in the evaluation of the patient, a good history and focal physical examination in the primary care setting can usually reveal the diagnosis.

In addition to diagnosing the patient, the goal of the primary clinician should be to recognize which patients need inpatient management or emergent intervention. This goal becomes particularly important when evaluating older patients. Several acute pathologic conditions can present with dizziness as the initial complaint. This article outlines the diagnostic approach to the dizzy patient, with emphasis on the differentiation of clinical emergencies.

---

* Corresponding author. Department of Emergency Medicine, Boston University Medical Center, One Boston Medical Center Place, Dowling One South, Boston, MA 02118.
 E-mail address: nchawla99@yahoo.com (N. Chawla).

Diagnostic approach

History

Obtaining a good history is the most critical step in the assessment of the dizzy patient. Because the term *dizzy* is used by patients to describe a variety of experiences, it is important to clarify the patient's actual complaint. The sensation of movement or spinning is classic for true vertigo. These patients may complain of objects moving around them (objective vertigo) or that they are spinning relative to their surroundings (subjective vertigo). Other patients may describe light-headedness or weakness. These symptoms should guide the clinician to investigate more systemic diseases consistent with presyncope.

Often, a good history can elicit whether a patient has true vertigo and whether the cause is central or peripheral. Vertigo, which is peripheral in origin, often presents as severe, intense attacks that last several seconds to minutes. Occasionally, more severe episodes last up to several hours and are accompanied by nausea, vomiting, and disequilibrium. Vertigo triggered by a change in position is also suggestive of a peripheral disorder. A central etiology is more concerning in patients who describe mild symptoms that are gradual in onset and last several weeks to months (Table 1).

It is also important for the physician to inquire about associated symptoms. Diseases of the middle and inner ear can cause hearing loss, aural fullness, and tinnitus along with vertigo. The physician should attempt to localize the auditory symptoms to one side. The symptomatic ear is often the one with vestibular damage. Associated neurologic symptoms are more consistent with central vertigo. Headaches may suggest dizziness associated with migraines. Other symptoms suggestive of a central disorder include visual changes, seizures, ataxia, or other gait disturbances. The presence of these symptoms should provoke further investigation and imaging.

A thorough medication history should also be reviewed. Several drugs are directly ototoxic and should be discontinued in any patient complaining of vertigo. These drugs include certain aminoglycosides, furosemide,

Table 1
Characteristics of peripheral and central vertigo

Characteristic	Peripheral	Central
Severity	Severe	Mild
Onset	Sudden	Gradual
Duration	Seconds to minutes	Weeks to months
Positional	Yes	No
Fatigable	Yes	No
Associated symptoms	Auditory	Neurologic and visual
Associated nystagmus	Horizontal	Vertical

ethacrynic acid, acetylsalicyclic acid, amiodarone, quinine, and cisplatinum. Psychotropic medications are also notorious for causing light-headedness and disequilibrium (Box 1), of which the most commonly encountered are anti-Alzheimer's medications, anticonvulsants, antidepressants, and anxiolytics. In addition, chronic use of vestibular suppressants such as meclizine and scopolamine may result in sensitization. Patients can have severe withdrawal symptoms when these medications are discontinued. A variety of medications can induce toxic labyrinthitis. In these cases, the offending medication should be immediately discontinued.

A complete social history is also important in patients complaining of dizziness. Alcohol, nicotine, and caffeine can all exacerbate vertiginous symptoms. Current or previous use of illicit drugs should be documented. Sexual history should also be noted. Certain sexually transmitted diseases such as syphilis have otologic symptoms. In addition, any history of traumatic head injury or cervical trauma should be investigated. Finally, it is important to remember that depression and anxiety can also manifest as dizziness.

Physical examination

After a good history has been obtained, the next important step is a thorough physical examination. Particular emphasis should be placed on the ocular examination. It is important to test pupillary reactivity and extraocular movements. Subtle ocular abnormalities can sometimes be the only clue to cerebellar disease. A fundoscopic examination should always be performed.

Box 1. Psychotropic medications that may cause dizziness

Anti-Alzheimer's (memantine, rivastigmine, tacrine)
Antipsychotics
- Typicals (chlorpromazine, prochlorperazine, fluphenazine, perphenazine, thioridazine, trifluoperazine)
- Atypicals (all except olanzapine)

Antidepressants
- Selective serotonin reuptake inhibitors (all)
- Tricyclics (amitriptyline, nortriptyline, trazodone, imipramine)
- Monoamine oxidase inhibitors (selegiline, phenelzine)
- Others (nefazodone, venlafaxine, mirtazapine, bupropion)

Anxiolytics (alprazolam, clonazepam, diazepam, lorazepam, oxazepam, chlordiazepoxide)
Mood stabilizers (gabapentin, carbamazepine, oxcarbazepine, lamotrigine)
Anticonvulsants (phenytoin)

Papilledema usually presents bilaterally and is indicative of elevated intracranial pressure. In these patients, vision is usually is well preserved and visual acuity testing does not offer significant additional information.

In patients who have unilateral vestibular disorders, horizontal beating nystagmus may be observed away from the side of the lesion. The abnormal jerk nystagmus that is classical for inner ear disease consists of slow and quick components. Patients exhibiting coarse vertical nystagmus may have a central lesion which is thought to be related to asymmetric vestibular input from both sides. Patients who have peripheral vestibular disease should be able to suppress the nystagmus by focusing their vision on a stationary target. The inability to suppress the nystagmus is suggestive of a central abnormality. It is often helpful to ask the patient's family whether they noted any unusual eye movements during the acute vertiginous episode which is particularly important with pediatric patients [2].

If nystagmus is not present at rest, then positional testing should be performed. The patient's eye movement should be noted while lying supine with the head extended and turned to one side. The test should be repeated with the head turned to the other side. Positional nystagmus is strongly suggestive of vestibular disease. This maneuver often reproduces vertiginous symptoms in patients who have a peripheral disorder. Because of the risk of dislodging atheromatous plaques in the vertebrobasilar vessels with sudden turning movements, this maneuver should be avoided in elderly patients.

When examining the ear, the clinician should use an otoscope to look for impacted cerumen or any foreign object in the ear canal. Often, removal of the foreign body relieves the symptoms of vertigo. It is also important to recognize signs of middle ear disease such as fluid behind the eardrum, perforation, or extensive scarring. The patient should be tested for any subtle hearing loss. If the hearing is abnormal, the Rinne and the Weber's tuning-fork tests can help determine whether the hearing loss is conductive or sensorineural.

The heart and carotid arteries should be auscultated because occasionally, a positive finding points to vascular causes of dizziness. Examinations significant for a carotid bruit, heart murmur, or irregular rhythm should impress upon the physician the need for a cardiovascular work-up. This work-up is particularly important in older patients or those who are at high risk for cerebrovascular disease.

A thorough neurologic examination is important in patients complaining of dizziness. A complete cranial nerve evaluation may help localize lesions of the midbrain, pons, and medulla. The patient's cerebellar function can be assessed with finger-to-nose pointing and rapidly alternating movements. Romberg's test is also useful in assessing the dizzy patient. The patient is asked to stand with feet together and arms folded. The inability to maintain posture in this position is suggestive of abnormal proprioception.

Any gait abnormality should arouse suspicion of a central lesion. The main features of an ataxic gait consistent with cerebellar disease are a wide base, unsteadiness, irregularity of steps, tremor of the trunk, and lurching from side to side. This unsteadiness is most prominent on arising quickly from sitting, turning sharply, and stopping suddenly while walking.

Laboratory tests

Most routine testing is not helpful in the evaluation of the patient who has vertiginous symptoms; however, in the absence of clinical findings or in the evaluation of the patient who has near syncope, a complete blood count and chemistry panel can be helpful. Some clinicians also recommend thyroid function tests, fasting glucose, and rheumatoid factor [3].

Electrocardiography

Because myocardial ischemia can present atypically in many patients, it is important to obtain an ECG on those patients who are older or have significant cardiac risk factors. In addition, any patient who requires an emergency room evaluation after being seen in the outpatient office should have an ECG reviewed before transfer.

Electronystagmography

Electronystagmography is an examination that records eye movements in response to vestibular, visual, cervical, caloric, rotational, and positional stimulation [4]. Electrodes are placed at the outer and inner canthi for horizontal recordings and above and below the eye for vertical recordings. Electronystagmography testing is helpful in assessing vestibular dysfunction but is limited in diagnosing nonvestibular disorders [5].

Radiologic imaging

When cerebellar hemorrhage, cerebellar infarction, or other central lesions are suspected, an emergent CT or MRI of the brain is indicated. These patients should be immediately transferred to an emergency department that has neuroimaging capabilities.

In patients at particularly high risk for cerebrovascular disease, magnetic resonance angiography can be used to visualize the intracranial vasculature. Although a less sensitive study than cerebral angiography because of its limited visualization of small vessels, magnetic resonance angiography remains more readily used by neurologists to evaluate high-risk patients.

MRI with gadolinium enhancement is particularly useful in detecting smaller intracanalicular tumors such as acoustic neuromas. It is also recommended for identifying sclerotic and demyelinating white matter lesions characteristic of multiple sclerosis. Although not indicated in younger patients who have a clear peripheral cause, radiologic imaging should be considered in all patients who have new-onset vertigo or neurologic findings [6,7].

Peripheral vertigo

Peripheral causes of vertigo arise from abnormalities in the vestibular end organs (semicircular canals and utricle), the vestibular nerve, and the vestibular nuclei. Most of these causes are benign and readily treatable.

Benign paroxysmal positional vertigo

The most common cause of peripheral vertigo is benign paroxysmal positional vertigo (BPPV). As the name implies, this condition is paroxysmal (sudden onset) and positional. Most patients report attacks provoked by turning their head. BPPV is characterized by its fatigability. The patient develops a tolerance to head movements, leading to a reduction in symptoms.

The condition occurs when debris (otoconia) from the utricle circulates within the endolymphatic system, causing positional irritation of the cupula and stimulating vertigo and nystagmus. Occasionally, the debris attaches to the cupula (cupulolithiasis) and symptoms persist for weeks.

The treatment of acute attacks of BPPV centers around symptomatic relief. Benzodiazepines, intravenously and orally, effectively relieve vertiginous symptoms because of their sedative effect. Anticholinergics and antihistamines have also been shown to be helpful in alleviating symptoms by mediating the amount of acetylcholine involved in vestibular reactions. A short course of meclizine or diphenhydramine may resolve the vertiginous symptoms. Antiemetics such as promethazine may improve the nausea associated with vertigo.

Canolith repositioning procedures treat BPPV by directing the otoconia back to the utricle where it is absorbed. The Epley and Semont maneuvers have been shown to be 85% to 95% effective in treating patients who have BPPV [8–10]; however, in more than half of patients, a recurrence of symptoms occurs [11]. In these cases, patient education and reassurance are important.

Otitis media

Patients who have otitis media often complain of vertigo. Because of the proximity of the vestibular end organs to the middle ear, the infectious process may extend to these structures. These patients are at risk for hearing loss and often end up with permanent labyrinthe deficits if left untreated. Extension of the infection into the mastoid can also occur, and these patients may develop an epidural abscess. With the early use of antibiotics and the treatment of the underlying otitis, these complications can usually be avoided.

Labyrinthitis

Labyrinthitis is a peripheral disorder characterized by inflammation of the canals of the inner ear. The cause of labyrinthitis is unknown, but because it commonly occurs following otitis media or an upper respiratory infection, it is thought to be a consequence of viral or bacterial infection [12]. It may also follow allergy, cholesteatoma, or the ingestion of certain drugs that are toxic to the inner ear. Patients who have acute labyrinthitis usually present with severe vertigo, hearing loss, nausea, vomiting, and fever.

Bacterial infections may directly invade the perilymphatic space, causing a suppurative labyrinthitis. These infections usually extend from the middle ear through a ruptured membrane or perilymph fistula. In patients who have meningitis, the infected cerebrospinal fluid enters the labyrinth through the cochlear aqueduct or internal auditory canal.

Patients who have bacterial labyrinthitis appear ill and require hospital admission and intravenous antibiotics. Occasionally, these patients also need surgical drainage and debridement. Bacterial labyrinthitis is one of the few causes of peripheral vertigo that requires early detection and transfer to the emergency department.

Vestibular neuritis

Vestibular neuritis usually results as a complication of an upper respiratory infection. The prevalence of vestibular neuritis peaks at age 40 to 50 years [13]. The virus affects the vestibular nuclei and causes sudden and severe vertigo, nausea, and vomiting. Auditory symptoms are usually absent. The diagnosis can be made on clinical presentation alone. Treatment with prednisone in the first 10 days of the attack may shorten the course of the illness. The acute attack is debilitating and patients often require bedrest.

Ramsay Hunt syndrome is caused by varicella zoster and is a variant of vestibular neuritis, with involvement of cranial nerves VII and VIII. It causes facial paresis, tinnitus, hearing loss, and a vestibular defect [14]. Patients who have Ramsay Hunt syndrome respond well to early initiation of prednisone and acyclovir.

Cholesteatoma

Cholesteatoma is a benign skin growth that occurs in the middle ear behind the ear drum. It is usually due to repeated infection, which causes an ingrowth of the skin of the eardrum. Over time, the cholesteatoma can increase in size and destroy the surrounding delicate bones of the middle ear. When this benign tumor erodes into the labyrinthe, it causes hearing loss and vertigo. The vertigo tends to be severe in these patients but typically does not last beyond a few seconds. Surgical removal of the cholesteastoma is indicated in symptomatic patients.

Trauma

The incidence of dizziness and dysequilibrium following head or neck injury is between 40% and 60%, even following mild or moderate head injuries not requiring acute hospitalization [15]. Any evidence of significant traumatic injury should incite a complete trauma evaluation [16]. Blunt head injury can concuss the membranous labyrinth with preservation of the otic capsule. Patients may complain of mild vertigo, disequilibrium, and nausea [17]. Symptoms tend to resolve spontaneously over several days to weeks.

Explosive blasts can also result in symptoms of vertigo. Pressure waves classically injure the ear by rupturing the tympanic membrane and disrupting the ossicular chain. The cochlea and hair cells can shear off the basilar membrane, causing significant inner ear damage.

Barotrauma to the inner ear is rare. It results from acute changes in atmospheric pressure. Deep-sea divers and pilots are particularly at risk for this type of injury. A perilymphatic fistula occurs when there is rupture of the oval or round windows that separate the perilymphatic space from the middle ear. Patients who have perilymphatic fistulas from barotrauma usually complain of a sudden onset of vertigo or dizziness. Patients are put on bedrest for 1 to 2 weeks and instructed to avoid any activities that would produce Valsalva-type maneuvers. Most patients heal spontaneously, but surgical repair is recommended in severe cases.

Endolymphatic hydrops

The most common form of endolymphatic hydrops is Meniere's disease. Patients may present with the classic triad of tinnitus, fluctuant sensorineural hearing loss, and vertigo. The vertigo attacks may last several minutes to an hour. It is not typical for these attacks to persist longer than several hours. As the disease progresses, attacks occur more frequently and are more severe. Although the disease starts unilaterally, almost half of patients develop bilateral auditory symptoms.

The predominant pathology of Meniere's disease is dilation of the endolymphatic system caused by excess production of endolymph or decreased reabsorption. Because salt in the diet is thought to increase the endolymphatic volume, the cornerstone of medical treatment involves salt restriction and diuretics. Greater than 90% of patients respond well to medical management [18]. For patients in whom medical therapy is not effective, surgical options include endolymphatic sac decompression or shunting, vestibular nerve resection, or labyrinthectomy. Chemical ablation of the vestibular apparatus has also gained wide acceptance as a treatment modality. In these cases, gentamycin is injected transtympanically. Although a less aggressive approach than surgery, chemical ablation has a greater risk of hearing loss.

Acoustic neuroma

An acoustic neuroma is a tumor composed of the Schwann cells of the vestibular nerve. Although vertigo is the most common presenting symptom, it is often associated with unilateral hearing loss or tinnitus [19]. In patients who have suspected acoustic neuroma, a gadolinium-enhanced MRI should be ordered. The MRI detects intracanalicular abnormalities with 100% sensitivity and is the "gold standard" for detecting this tumor. Because there is a potential for the tumor to expand intracranially, the patient should be reimaged regularly [20,21]. Treatment options include radiotherapy or surgical removal.

Central vertigo

Central vertigo manifests as marked vertigo, nausea, and vertical nystagmus. Neurologic symptoms such as headache or gait ataxia may also be present. In severe cases, patients may have depressed levels of consciousness. The cerebellum is often involved, and etiologies include multiple sclerosis, tumor, hemorrhage, and ischemia. Vascular injuries and infarcts of the central neurologic system can cause permanent debilitating disease. Because central processes have more serious consequences, aggressive work-up and treatment are recommended.

Even in patients who have mild symptoms, it is important to maintain a high level of clinical suspicion when advanced age, atrial fibrillation, hypertension, or previous cerebrovascular disease is present. Often, vertigo is the only presenting symptom in patients who have impending infarction. When a central etiology is suspected, the patient should be transferred immediately by ambulance to an emergency department for neurologic imaging. Evaluation by neurology and neurosurgery may be needed.

Cerebellar hemorrhage

In patients who have acute neurologic deficit, it is often difficult to distinguish intracranial hemorrhage from ischemic infarct. It is imperative not to administer anticoagulant medicine, including aspirin, until intracranial hemorrhage has been ruled out by imaging. Because the posterior fossa is a relatively small and nonexpandable space, hemorrhage can lead to rapid compression and compromise of vital medullary functions, obstructive hydrocephalus, or herniation of the medullary tonsils. Endotracheal intubation may be needed to protect the airway, control breathing, and allow therapeutic hyperventilation. Because neurosurgical consultation may be needed for surgical decompression by way of suboccipital craniectomy or ventriculostomy, all patients who have a presentation of central disease should be transferred only to centers that have neurosurgical capabilities.

Brainstem ischemia

Vertigo may occur from infarcts in the posterior fossa that contain vestibular pathways. The cerebellar circulation is complex, and it is often difficult to localize the area of ischemia without magnetic resonance angiography.

The anterior inferior cerebellar artery divides into several branches that perfuse the lateral cerebellum, the pons, and the labyrinth. Several types of anterior inferior cerebellar artery syndromes result in acute vertigo. Infarct of the anterior vestibular artery can present with peripheral symptoms only. Infarct of the common cochlear artery causes peripheral symptoms and hearing loss and tinnitus. Patients who have infarcts of the pontine branch can present with central signs such as dysarthria, facial palsy, sensory loss, Horner syndrome, and dysmetria [22].

The posterior inferior cerebellar artery perfuses part of the cerebellum and the dorsolateral medulla. Infarcts in the lateral medulla often damage the vestibular nucleus and cause vertigo. This condition is known as Wallenberg syndrome and characterized by crossed sensory signs, ipsilateral lateropulsion, ataxia, and Horner's sign.

Vertebrobasilar insufficiency

Vertebrobasilar insufficiency occurs when there is narrowing of the arteries that supply the posterior brain (subclavian, vertebral, or basilar arteries). It is usually the result of hardening of the arteries (atherosclerosis) and occurs among patients older than 50 years. The narrowed arteries decrease the blood flow and, therefore, the oxygen to the vestibular center in the brain. Because the vestibular system is very sensitive to a lack of oxygen, difficulty with balance is often one of the first symptoms of vertebrobasilar insufficiency.

Transient ischemic attacks from vertebrobasilar ischemia provoke episodes of dizziness that are abrupt and usually last only a few minutes. They are frequently associated with other symptoms, most commonly visual disturbance, drop attacks, unsteadiness, or weakness. Changing or rapidly progressive symptoms should also raise suspicions of impending posterior circulation occlusion.

Vertebrobasilar insufficiency should be considered in any patient of advanced age who has new-onset vertigo without an obvious cause [6]. These patients should be evaluated by and admitted to the neurology service. Magnetic resonance arteriography can be performed to assess posterior circulation vessels and transcranial Doppler may detect decreased flow in the basilar artery. Treatment includes reduction of risk factors for cerebrovascular disease and antiplatelet therapy. Warfarin is used when there is significant vertebral or basilar artery stenosis [23]. Fig. 1 summarizes the management and disposition for patients who have central or peripheral vertigo.

Dizziness

In patients who complain of dizziness without clear vertiginous symptoms, the differential remains broad. Many patients complain of disequilibrium and imbalance, whereas others note light-headedness and other

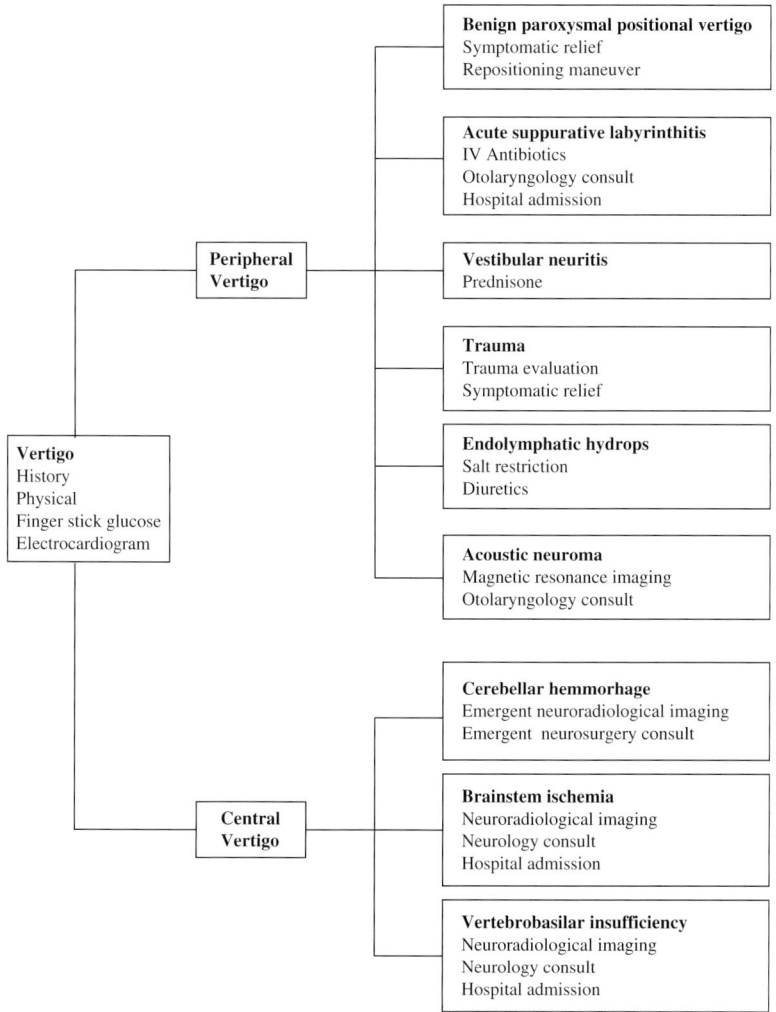

Fig. 1. Management of vertigo.

presyncope symptoms. Often, dizziness can be a multisensory disorder due to any combination of peripheral neuropathy, visual impairment, and musculoskeletal disease.

Proprioceptive abnormalities

Many diseases directly affect the proprioceptive sensory fibers. Chronic alcoholism is among the diseases manifesting with symptoms of dizziness and imbalance. These patients may have deterioration of the vestibulospinal pathways. These symptoms are usually not reversible and the patient must be counseled on safety and fall risk. Chronic alcoholism can also lead to compromised vitamin absorption from the gastrointestinal tract, leading to peripheral neurologic changes.

Syphilis is another rare but important cause of dizziness. In tertiary syphilis (tabes dorsalis), there is a deterioration of the posterior columns. These patients have compromised proprioception and often complain of difficulty walking in the dark.

Cerebral anoxia

A number of conditions can lead to poor blood flow to the central nervous system. These patients do not classically complain of light-headedness while sitting or lying down. Their symptoms can usually be reproduced with standing. Anemia may produce cerebral anoxia and can result from any number of causes. Iron deficiency, malignancy, vitamin deficiency, and chronic blood loss are some examples. Patients who have significant arteriosclerosis may also complain of positional symptoms. In these patients, other neurologic symptoms including weakness and syncope may be present.

Orthostatic hypotension is often seen in patients who complain of dizziness when arising to a standing position. The symptoms are generally transient and resolve spontaneously. In these cases, medication-induced hypotension must be ruled out. Often, no underlying cause is found for the autonomic response.

Metabolic disorders

Many patients who have thyroid dysfunction can present with dizziness as an initial complaint. Many patients also have dizziness associated with pregnancy or menstruation. It has been well documented that acute changes in hormone levels commonly lead to symptoms of light-headedness. Hypoglycemia can also cause dizziness. In patients who do not have an obvious diagnosis, a finger-stick blood glucose should be performed [24].

Migraines

The mechanism of dizziness or vertigo from migraines is unknown. Migraine is a vascular disease characterized by periodic, unilateral headaches. These headaches are often preceded for a variable time by associated neurologic symptoms called the aura. In individuals who have migraine, dizziness and vertigo can occur as part of the aura or separately. Spells usually last approximately an hour but can last several hours or days in patients who have severe symptoms. Most patients who have migraines have a long history of recurring symptoms.

The management of migraine is divided into two categories: symptomatic and preventive treatments. Acute attacks can be treated with various nonopioid analgesics. Preventive treatment is most frequently accomplished with amitryptiline, β-blockers, calcium channel blockers, and acetazolamide.

Acetazolamide has been particularly effective in treating patients who have vestibular symptoms associated with migraine.

Presyncope

Presyncopal patients complain of feeling faint and light-headed without losing consciousness. Sometimes nausea, dizziness, diaphoresis, and a sense of warmth accompany a feeling of faintness. Patients who have a history of unexplained fainting or recurring presyncope often need an inpatient evaluation to investigate cardiac causes of their symptoms. The work-up and treatment of these patients is discussed more thoroughly in articles on syncope.

Psychogenic

Psychogenic dizziness often occurs in patients who have chronic anxiety. The complaints are often vague, numerous, and out of proportion to the physical findings. In other patients, panic attacks manifest as sudden intense fear or discomfort and reach a crescendo within 10 minutes. They are frequently associated with brief episodes of dizziness, nausea, shortness of breath, chest tightness, paresthesias, and diaphoresis. Physical examination findings in patients who have psychogenic disorders are often dramatic. They include excessive slowness or hesitation, exaggerated sway on standing, and sudden buckling of the knees.

Selective serotonin reuptake inhibitors are the mainstay of treatment for panic disorders and chronic anxiety. Counseling and behavior modification are also frequently helpful.

Summary

Dizziness and vertigo present in patients of all ages. Particularly in older patients, dizziness is associated with a variety of cardiovascular, neurosensory, and psychiatric conditions and with the use of multiple medications [25]. For the patient, the symptoms can be debilitating. In patients older than 60 years, 20% have experienced dizziness severe enough to affect their daily activities [26]. Appropriate diagnosis and treatment can significantly improve quality of life. Most causes of dizziness are benign, but early recognition of serious or life-threatening disease is important. Management of these patients includes referral for neuroimaging and further evaluation in an emergency department.

References

[1] Kroenke K, Mangelsdorff D. Common symptoms in ambulatory care incidence, evaluation, therapy, and outcome. Am J Med 1989;86:262–6.

[2] Eviatar L. Dizziness in children. Otolaryngol Clin North Am 1994;27:557–71.
[3] Paydarfar JA, Goebel JA. Integrated clinical and laboratory vestibular evaluation. Curr Curr Opin Otolaryngol Head Neck Surg 2000;8:363–8.
[4] American Academy of Neurology. Assessment: electronystagmography. Report of the Therapeutics and Technology Assessment Subcommittee. Neurology 1996;46:1763–6.
[5] Baloh RW, Honrubia V. Clinical neurophysiology of the vestibular system. 2nd edition. Philadelphia: FA Davis; 1990.
[6] Fife TD, Baloh RW, Duckwiler GR. Isolated dizziness in vertebrobasilar insufficiency: clinical features, angiography, and follow-ups. J Stroke Cerebrovasc Dis 1994;4:4–12.
[7] Gizzi M, Riley E, Molinari S. The diagnostic value of imaging the patient with dizziness: a Bayesian approach. Arch Neurol 1996;53:1299–304.
[8] Fung K, Hall SF. Particle repositioning maneuver: effective treatment for benign paroxysmal positional vertigo. J Otolaryngol 1996;25:243–8.
[9] Koelliker P, Summers R, Hawkins B. Benign paroxysmal positional vertigo: diagnosis and treatment in the emergency department—a review of the literature and discussion of canalith-repositioning maneuvers. Ann Emerg Med 2001;37(4):392–8.
[10] Yimantae K, Srirompotong S, Srirompotong S, et al. A randomized trial of the canalith repositioning procedure. Laryngoscope 2003;113(5):828–32.
[11] Wolf JS, Boyev KP, Manokey BJ, et al. Success of the modified Epley maneuver in treating benign paroxysmal vertigo. Laryngoscope 1999;109:900–3.
[12] Paparella MM, Goycoolen MV, Meyerhoff WL. Inner ear pathology and otitis media: a review. Anal Otol Rhinyl Laryngol 1980;89:249–53.
[13] Sekitani T, Imate Y, Noguchi T, et al. Vestibular neuronitis: epidemiological survey by questionnaire in Japan. Act Otololaryngol Suppl 1993;503:85–9.
[14] Adour KK. Otological complications of herpes zoster. Ann Neurol 1994;35:S62–4.
[15] Wennmo C, Svensson C. Temporal bone fractures. Vestibular and other ear related sequelae. Acta Otolaryngol Suppl 1989;468:379–83.
[16] Mallinson AI, Longridge NS. Dizziness from whiplash and head injuries: differences between whiplash and head injury. Am J Otol 1998;19:814–8.
[17] Schessel DA, Nedzalski JM. Meniere's disease and other peripheral vestibular disorders. In: Otololaryngology–head and neck surgery. St Louis (MO): Mosby-Year Book; 1993. p. 3168–71.
[18] Shinkawa H, Kimura RD. Effect of diuretics on endolymphatic hydrops. Acta Otolaryngol 1986;101:43–52.
[19] Deen HG, Ebersold MJ, Harner SG, et al. Conservative management of acoustic neuroma: an outcome study. Neurosurgery 1996;39:260–4.
[20] Mirz F, Jorgenson B, Fiirgaard B, et al. Investigations into the natural history of vestibular schwannomas. Clin Otolaryngol 1999;24:13–8.
[21] Pollock BE, Lunsford LD, Kondziolka D, et al. Vestibular schwannomas management. J Neurosurg 1998;89:949–55.
[22] Oas JG, Baloh RW. Vertigo and the anterior inferior cerebellar artery syndrome. Neurology 1992;42:2274–9.
[23] Gomez CR, Cruz-Flores S, Malkoff S, et al. Isolated vertigo as a manifestation of vertebrobasilar ischemia. Neurology 1996;47:94–7.
[24] Herr RD, Zun L, Mathews JJ. A directed approach to the dizzy patient. Ann Emerg Med 1989;18:664–72.
[25] Sloan P, Coeytaux R, Beck R, et al. Dizziness: state of the science. Ann Internal Med 2001;134(9 part 2):823–32.
[26] Lawson J, Fitzgerald J, Birchall J, et al. Diagnosis of geriatric patients with severe dizziness. J Am Geriatr Soc 1999;47:113.

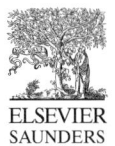

Approach to Ophthalmologic Emergencies

Jerry Naradzay, MD[a,1], Robert A. Barish, MD[b,*]

[a]*Emergency Medical Services, Mesa View Regional Hospital, Mesquite, NV, USA*
[b]*Office of the Dean, University of Maryland School of Medicine, Baltimore, MD, USA*

Primary care practitioners must be familiar with ophthalmologic emergencies because eye injuries, medical conditions, infections, and vision-threatening conditions affect infants, children, adults, and the elderly. Infants are susceptible to ophthalmia neonatorum, or infant conjunctivitis, including *Chlamydia* conjunctivitis, a vision-threatening infection. Infants, children, and teenagers are at risk for vision loss from arterial obstruction, optic neuritis, chemical injury, or direct globe trauma. Each year, the 20- to 34-year-old age group sustains almost 300,000 work-related eye injuries that require emergency treatment [1]. It is estimated that one of every 20 elderly people, nearly 3% of whites and more than 3% of blacks [2], experience a visual loss that affects their daily living [3]. Medical conditions such as macular degeneration, cataracts, diabetic retinopathy, and glaucoma are the primary causes of ophthalmologic conditions in this group.

This article presents evaluation and treatment approaches to ophthalmologic conditions that are likely to be encountered in a primary care office, which can be organized by diagnostic category, symptoms, and location of complaint (Box 1). By using one or a combination of these categories, the practitioner can provide appropriate, timely, and effective ophthalmology evaluation and treatment. Acute conditions are categorized in Box 2 according to the urgency of intervention.

In preparation for evaluating and treating patients with ophthalmologic conditions, the health care provider must establish a good relationship with an ophthalmologist and optometrist for patients who require a specialist's intervention. The primary practitioner and eye specialist can discuss

---

* Corresponding author. Clinical Affairs, University of Maryland School of Medicine, 655 West Baltimore Street, 14th Floor, Baltimore, MD 21201, USA.
    E-mail address: rbarish@som.umaryland.edu (R.A. Barish).
[1] *Present address:* Emergency Services, Maria Parham Medical Center, Henderson, NC.

Box 1. Methods of organizing ophthalmologic conditions

Diagnostic category
1. True emergencies
   - Central retinal artery occlusion (CRAO)
   - Alkali burn
2. Loss of vision
   - Sudden
     - Central retinal vein occlusion (CRVO)
     - Lens dislocation
   - Progressive
3. Blunt trauma (location)
4. Penetrating trauma (location)
   - Lid
   - Muscle
   - Lacrimal system
   - Cornea
     - Foreign body
     - Laceration
     - Penetration
   - Globe
   - Anterior chamber
   - Lens
   - Posterior chamber
   - Retina
   - Vasculature
   - Bony orbit
5. Chemical exposure
6. Red eye
   - Viral
   - Bacterial
   - Allergic
7. Vascular injury
8. Lacrimation disorders
9. Extraocular movement disorders

Symptom
1. Vision loss
   - Painless
   - Painful
2. Double vision
3. Trauma
4. Chemical exposure
5. Red eye and discharge
6. Eye pain

> *Location*
> 1. Extraocular and periorbital
> 2. Sclera
> 3. Cornea
> 4. Anterior chamber
> 5. Lens
> 6. Posterior chamber
> 7. Retina
> 8. Vascular

indications for referral, specific interventions, treatments, and diagnostic plans, such as when to

- patch the eye;
- initiate topical steroid therapy;
- initiate cycloplegic therapy and the type of medication to use;
- measure intraocular pressure in the primary physician's office;
- make a same-day referral;
- make an urgent (2- to 3-day) referral;
- make a routine referral (within 7 days); and
- order ultrasonography, a CT scan, or a MRI scan.

Ophthalmic equipment required for office-based evaluation and intervention includes

- a wall-mounted and handheld Snellen visual acuity chart for adults and children;
- direct ophthalmoscope;
- fluorescein strip paper;
- cobalt light source;
- ophthalmic medications (see Box 3);
- lens irrigation system, such as intravenous tubing and sterile saline bags, a Morgan lens, or an eye wash; station
- eye patches;
- tonometer; and
- slit lamp (required for practitioners who intend to examine the cornea and anterior chamber, measure intraocular pressure, and remove corneal foreign bodies).

Primary care physicians should educate patients as appropriate about common eye disorders and have relevant patient education materials readily available. Topics can include symptoms of glaucoma, ocular infections, elevated intraocular pressure, macular degeneration, dry eye syndrome, and instructions about what to do if the eye is injured.

> **Box 2. Acute ophthalmic conditions**
>
> *Emergency*
>   Alkali burns
>   Retinal arterial occlusion
>
> *Very urgent*
>   Acute angle closure glaucoma
>   Globe perforation
>   Globe rupture
>
> *Urgent*
>   Corneal abrasion
>   Corneal ulcer
>   Hyphema
>   Intraocular foreign body
>   Macular edema
>   Orbital cellulitis
>   Orbital injury
>   Retinal detachment

The physician should also ensure that patients have an accurate list of ophthalmic and systemic medications [4] and know how to administer them (Box 3).

Workplace injuries occur at a rate of approximately 1000 per day. Therefore, the primary care physician should ensure that patients who are at risk for eye injury during the workday or while engaging in hobbies or sports have the proper corrective lens and use protective measures [5]. Eye injury risks are listed in Box 4.

Central retinal artery occlusion

CRAO and alkali burns are true eye emergencies because seconds count in the prevention of vision loss or impairment. Occlusion time, cause, and the patency of the cilioretinal artery are factors that influence macular viability and vision loss [6]. Retinal blood flow must be restored within 90 minutes for vision to be preserved [7]. Typically, the patient who presents with CRAO is a 50- to 70-year-old with a sudden painless vision loss, which often occurs between midnight and 6 AM, less often between 6 AM and noon. Although retinal artery occlusion is caused typically by embolization from a cardiac or vascular source, it is a rare condition [8]. However, it is important to keep in mind that numerous conditions and interventions can cause retinal artery obstruction (Box 5).

Box 3. Guidelines for the prescription and use of ophthalmic medications

1. When treating a patient with bacterial or viral conjunctivitis, do not patch the eye.
2. Before prescribing ophthalmic medication, perform a complete medication review.
3. Review the drug interactions and systemic side effects associated with ophthalmic medications.
4. Provide topical or systemic pain medication.
5. Administer solutions and liquids at least 10 minutes after administering topical ophthalmic gel medication.
6. Instruct the patient on the proper technique for administering topical ophthalmic medication:
   - Wash hands thoroughly before and after applying medication
   - Hold the bottle or dispensing tube in the hand opposite to the affected eye
   - With the lid on the bottle, invert it and shake it once
   - Use the fingers on the hand on the same side as the affected eye to pull down the lower eyelid by pulling on the skin above the cheekbone
   - Tilt the head back
   - Squeeze the bottle to place the required number of drops onto the pocket formed by the lower lid; do not let the bottle tip touch the eye
   - Close the eyelid
   - Gently depress the fleshy part on the side of the eye near the nose bridge (this prevents the medication from washing out too rapidly)
   - Wash hands after applying the medication
   - Store the medication at room temperature and away from children
7. Instruct the patient to bring the medication when going to the emergency department or to the ophthalmologist's or the primary care provider's office.

The signs of CRAO [31] are listed below.

- Visual acuity is limited to light perception or counting fingers.
- Afferent pupillary defect or Marcus Gunn pupil
- The retina appears white because of intracellular edema, except at the fovea, where it is thin, and the choroid shows, giving a "cherry red spot" (not pathognomic).

Box 4. Exposures that increase the risk of eye injury

Blood and body fluids
Chemicals such as acids, bases, fuels, solvents, and lime
Dust, concrete, metal, and other particles
Falling or shifting debris, building materials, and glass
Smoke and noxious or poisonous gases
Thermal hazards and fires
Ultraviolet light
Welding light and electrical arcs
Wet or dry cement powder

- Cholesterol plaque: yellow Hollenhorst plaques may be seen at an arteriole bifurcation.
- Narrowing and irregularities of the arterioles and venules
- Central vision may be spared if the macular bundle is supplied by the cilioretinal artery.

Treatment must be initiated quickly to lower intraocular pressure (IOP) and restore blood flow to the retina within 90 to 100 minutes from the time

Box 5. Causes of retinal artery occlusion

Associated with medical conditions
   Systemic lupus erythematosus [9,10]
   Giant cell arteritis [11,12]
   Acute lymphoblastic leukemia [13]
   Internal carotid artery dissection [14]
   Primary central nervous system vasculitis [15]
   Homocystinemia [16]
   Patent foramen ovale [17]
   Orbital pseudotumor [18,19]
   Iron deficiency anemia [20]
   Posterior scleritis [21]
   Fibromuscular dysplasia [22]
   Wegener's granulomatosis [23,24]

As a complication
   Blunt ocular trauma [25]
   Coronary angiography [26]
   Embolization of a maxillary sinus tumor [27]
   Laryngectomy [28]
   Spinal surgery [29]
   Peribulbar anesthesia [30]

of occlusion (not from the time the patient presents for evaluation). The often-quoted 90-minute window is based on the results of numerous experimental studies [7,32]. The clinical "pearl" is that the intervention window is narrow and therefore treatment must be initiated decisively.

Interventions include the application of oral acetylsalicylate, oral acetazolamide, ocular massage, isovolemic hemodilution, oral pentoxifylline, topical β-blocker, paracentesis of the anterior chamber, subcutaneous heparin, selective retinal artery infusion with a thrombolytic agent, and hyperbaric oxygen treatment. Each procedure has proponents and detractors [33]. Systemic corticosteroids are needed when central retinal artery occlusion has been caused by arteritis [34,35]. The practitioner must choose, in conjunction with the patient and ophthalmologist, the best intervention plan. As with any intervention, the procedure should not cause harm, should be beneficial, and should be initiated immediately.

Immediate treatment is massaging the globe for 15 minutes. Pharmacologic treatment to lower IOP is the next step. Topical, oral, and intravenous medications can be administered while the globe is being massaged. Anterior chamber paracentesis, administered through an anesthetized cornea, can lower the pressure, but this procedure requires specialized training.

A promising intervention for restoring retinal blood flow is selective infusion of the ophthalmic artery or vein with a thrombolytic agent [8,34]. The practicability of this intervention must be determined well in advance of treating the first patient with an ophthalmic vascular insult. The practitioner is encouraged to develop emergency plans with a local interventional radiology service and ophthalmologist for evaluating and treating central retinal artery or vein occlusion. Similarly, if hyperbaric oxygen treatment will be considered for some ophthalmologic conditions, the practitioner must know where this intervention can be performed and by whom [36].

Retrobulbar neuritis

Retrobulbar neuritis requires urgent intervention. It is a form of optic neuritis in which the optic nerve becomes inflamed. It can be idiopathic or caused by infections such as meningitis, syphilis, Lyme disease, and viral illnesses. Noninfectious causes include multiple sclerosis, tumors, exposure to chemicals, and allergic reactions. Vision loss can range from minimal to complete blindness. The average age of people who develop optic neuritis is 32. The typical presentation of optic neuritis is a woman in her early 30s complaining of blurred vision, loss of central vision (scotoma), colors that appear dull ("wash out"), pain with eye movement, and a tender eye. Retrobulbar neuritis can be an early sign of multiple sclerosis. Up to 40% of the 25,000 people who develop optic neuritis in the United States each year will develop multiple sclerosis within 10 years [37].

Optic neuritis usually affects only one eye but can involve both eyes. In the early stages of retrobulbar neuritis, the optic disk appears normal. In later stages, a pale disk is common. The pupillary response to light can be reduced in the affected eye. Retrobulbar optic neuritis secondary to varicella zoster infection should be considered in immunocompromised patients, even in the absence of cutaneous or retinal lesions [38].

Emergency consultation with an ophthalmologist is required to decide on the therapeutic plan, notably the dosage, duration, and type of steroid therapy. Cases in which there is no obvious cause or in which the cause is multiple sclerosis often improve after 2 weeks, but the vision may never completely return to normal.

Alkali burns

Alkaline burns of the eye are more severe than acid burns because of the rapid penetration through the cornea and anterior chamber, combining with cell membrane lipids, causing disruption of the cells and stromal mucopolysaccharides with concomitant tissue softening [39]. The release of collagenases and proteases after the injury leads to corneoscleral melting [40]. Lye, cement cleaner, drain cleaner, fertilizer, sparklers, and firecrackers produce alkaline burns because they contain sodium hydroxide. Severe corneal liquefaction necrosis occurs after exposure to these agents.

Immediately after chemical injury, it is important to relieve the patient of pain. Systemic agents are often used to abort violent pain. The clinician must then estimate and grade the severity of limbal, conjunctival, and scleral ischemia and necrosis. The eye must be irrigated with copious amounts of water or saline. Irrigation should continue until the lacrimation fluid has a pH level between 6.8 and 7.4 [39,41]. An ophthalmologist must be involved in the initial evaluation and intervention for these patients.

Acid burns

Urgent treatment for acid burns should include prompt pain management and reassuring measures. Acid burns act quickly to cause coagulation necrosis of the corneal epithelium. Hydrofluoric acid exposes the corneum to fluoride ions, which quickly chelate calcium and magnesium [42]. Penetration and corneal damage may be limited by the formation of a coagulum. The patient requires assurance and emotional support. The amount of injury can range from reversible edema to stromal scarring, calcific band keratopathy, and iris and ciliary body fibrosis [43]. Treatment includes copious saline irrigation in addition to brisk pain management [43]. Irrigation with 1% calcium gluconate must be avoided [44]. The use of topical and intravenous antibiotics is controversial and should be discussed with an ophthalmologist.

Conjunctivitis and red eye

In conjunctivitis, the eye appears red because the blood vessels on the bulbar conjunctiva are engorged. The conjunctival eye can have a clear and watery or discolored and thick discharge, depending on the cause of the inflammation (eg, viral, bacterial, allergic or vernal, toxic, chemical, or parasitic [eg, *Chlamydia*]) (Tables 1 and 2). Each causative agent has distinguishing features and requires different treatments. The patient may complain of itching, heavy tearing, a gritty sensation, and crusting eyelids. With the exception of the allergic type, conjunctivitis is typically contagious.

Bacterial conjunctivitis can be a bilateral or unilateral condition. The lid and lashes may be covered with a mucopurulent discharge. Visual acuity is usually unaffected. Required treatments include warm compresses, irrigation when the patient showers, and the application of a broad-range topical antibiotic. In both bacterial and parasitic conjunctivitis (Table 3), visual acuity is usually not affected. Patching is discouraged.

Gonococcal conjunctivitis causes a purulent discharge associated with preauricular adenopathy. In neonates, it is usually bilateral and appears 3 to 5 days after vaginal delivery. Adults with gonococcal conjunctivitis are more likely to have a unilateral infection. Complications include ulcerative keratitis, visual loss, and corneal perforation [45]. The practitioner should be familiar with the antibiotic sensitivity profile for this and other sexually transmitted diseases. Intramuscular injections of penicillin or cephalosporin are effective for infections limited to the conjunctiva in adults [45]. Successful treatment has been reported from a single intramuscular dose of cefoxitin (2 g) and oral probenecid (1 g) [46] and from oral norfloxacin taken in a single dose or twice daily for 3 days [47]. The patient and the patient's at-risk contacts can also be treated with a single dose of intramuscular ceftriaxone (125 mg) followed by oral doxycycline (100 mg), taken twice daily for 7 days.

Chlamydial conjunctivitis is an intracellular infection of the inner lid. Performing an expanded history and physical examination is important for all eye infections but particularly when chlamydial conjunctivitis is suspected based on the patient's complaints of itching and an irritating mucous discharge that have lasted for several days or weeks. The provider must question the patient about sexual practices and exposure because chlamydial conjunctivitis is a disease of sexually active individuals. Women seem to be more susceptible to chlamydial infections than men are. The patient may also complain of symptoms of vaginitis or urethritis.

"Ophthalmia neonatorum" is a term for a condition that applies to acute conjunctivitis in the newborn from any cause. The infectious organisms are *Chlamydia trachomatis*, *Staphylococcus*, *Neisseria gonorrhoeae*,

Table 1
Features of conjunctivitis based on cause

Feature	Cause
Purulent discharge	Bacteria
Serous or clear discharge	Virus
Stringy, white discharge	Allergy
Preauricular lymphadenopathy	Virus (herpes simplex, *Gonococcus*)

Table 2
Comparison of the features and causes of red eye

Feature	Causes			
	Conjunctivitis	Iritis	Acute glaucoma	Keratitis (foreign body abrasion)
Discharge	Marked	None	None	Slight or none
Photophobia	None	Marked	Slight	Slight
Pain	None	Slight to marked	Marked	Marked
Visual acuity	Normal	Reduced	Reduced	Varies with site of lesion
Pupil	Normal	Smaller or same	Large and fixed	Smaller or same

Data from Birt C. The red eye. Faculty of Medicine, University of Toronto, 2001; with permission. Available at: http://eyelearn.med.utoronto.ca/Lectures04-05/RedEye/RedEyeChart.htm. Accessed July 18, 2005.

Streptococcus, *Haemophilus*, herpes simplex virus, molluscum contagiosum virus, and papillomavirus [48]. If *C trachomatis* is the offending organism, then the term is "*Chlamydia* ophthalmia neonatorum." *C trachomatis* infects infants as they pass through the birth canal if the mother has an untreated infection. Symptoms of conjunctivitis develop within the first 10 days of life. A child with ophthalmia neonatorum should be evaluated for lower respiratory chlamydial infection.

Staphylococcal allergic conjunctivitis presents with multiple ulcers at the limbus. The pathogenesis may be induced by an allergy to staphylococcal toxin. Treatment includes the topical application of 10% sulfacetamide or tobramycin. As with other bacterial infections, the eye should not be patched. An ophthalmologist may add a topical corticosteroid to the treatment regimen.

Viral conjunctivitis (Table 4) typically does not affect the patient's visual acuity. Patching is discouraged. Itching can be treated with nonsedating antihistamines. Epidemics are common. Viral conjunctivitis is difficult to distinguish from bacterial conjunctivitis on clinical grounds. Viral conjunctivitis is more frequently bilateral with ipsilateral preauricular adenopathy. Treatment includes the administration of a topical antiviral agent.

Table 3
Features and treatment of bacterial and parasitic conjunctivitis

Feature	Treatment			
	Bacterial	Gonococcal	Chlamydial	Staphylococcal
Laterality	Bi- or unilateral	Bilateral	Bilateral	Bilateral
Discharge	Mucopurulent discharge on lids and lashes	Purulent	Inclusion conjunctivitis within 14 d postpartum	Purulent
Prognosis	Good	Good	Good	Good
Treatment	Antimicrobial	Systemic penicillin, cephalosporin	Systemic and topical antimicrobial	Topical antimicrobial agent; consider steroid application

Table 4
Comparison of the features and treatment of viral, allergic and vernal, and vaccinia conjunctivitis

	Conjunctivitis		
Feature	Viral	Allergic and vernal	Vaccinia
Laterality	More frequently bilateral	Usually unilateral	Unilateral
Discharge	Mucopurulent discharge on lids and lashes	Inclusion conjunctivitis within 14 d postpartum	Papules, pustules, ulcerations, vesicles, mucopurulent drainage
Prognosis	Good	Good	—
Treatment	Antimicrobial	Antihistamines and topical decongestants	Topical trifluridine; consider vaccinia immunoglobulin
Chararcteristics	Preauricular adenopathy; contagious	Palpebral cobblestone papillae	History of contact with smallpox vaccine within 9 d preceding exposure

Keratoconjunctivitis describes the inflammation of the cornea in addition to the bulbar conjunctiva. Epidemic keratoconjunctivitis, a highly contagious form of viral conjunctivitis, is caused by adenovirus type 8. Individuals with this type of infection have tender ipsilateral preauricular nodes and subepithelial infiltrates. Epidemics are frequent. Contact with the cornea should be avoided. Ophthalmology referral is needed, as is a topical antibiotic to prevent secondary infection. Trifluorothymidine, a steroid, can be used in severe cases.

Allergic and vernal conjunctivitis are characterized by cobblestone papillae under the upper lid. Allergic reaction to an insect protein may cause marked chemosis and eye itching with symptoms out of proportion to findings. Distinct from a viral conjunctivitis, allergic conjunctivitis is usually uniocular. Treatment includes topical antihistamines, a vasoconstrictor, and the application of cool compresses.

Vaccinia conjunctivitis occurs after exposure to smallpox vaccine. "Kissing" lesions arise on opposing surfaces of the upper and lower lids. Treatment absolutely requires an ophthalmologic consultation. The local public health department must be contacted to consider treating the patient with hyperimmune globulin.

Scleritis

Scleritis is a painful, chronic inflammatory disease characterized by edema and cellular infiltration of the scleral and episcleral tissues. It has the potential to cause blindness [49]. The symptoms and treatment of scleritis are summarized in Table 5.

Scleritis can be classified as anterior and posterior, depending on its position on the globe in reference to the cornea. Anterior scleritis can be diffuse, nodular, or necrotizing, with or without inflammation (scleromalacia perforans). Necrotizing scleritis with or without inflammation is seen less frequently than the diffuse or nodular form but is more threatening to the

Table 5
Comparison of scleritis and episcleritis

Feature	Scleritis	Episcleritis
Symptom	Severe pain; visual symptoms	Painless; no visual symptoms
Patient age	> 50 y	20–50 y
Prognosis	Peripheral ulcerative keratitis with corneal perforation secondary glaucoma; scleral melting and perforation; exudative retinal detachment	Benign course
Phenylephrine response	No response	May blanch episcleral vessels
Treatment	Steroids; topical cyclosporine; scleral grafting	Reassurance; NSAIDs

vision. Posterior scleritis is characterized by flattening of the posterior aspect of the globe, thickening of the posterior coats of the eye (choroid and sclera), and retrobulbar edema.

All forms of scleritis cause severe pain, which occurs bilaterally more than 50% of the time and follows a gradual onset. Additional symptoms include a red, injected eye caused by inflamed vasculature. The patient may complain of tearing, photophobia, tenderness, and decreased visual acuity. Mucopurulent discharge is not a common feature, but it does occur in approximately 25% of patients with scleritis. The patient may have globe tenderness because structures are inflamed and swollen. A patient with scleritis has pain with eye movement or palpation, whereas a simple viral conjunctivitis does not have these features.

Scleritis is often associated with autoimmune conditions (eg, rheumatoid arthritis, systemic lupus erythematosus, ankylosing spondylitis, Reiter syndrome, psoriatic arthritis, gouty arthritis, inflammatory bowel diseases, relapsing polychondritis, polymyositis, Sjögren's syndrome, mixed connective tissue disease, and progressive systemic sclerosis). The autoimmune inflammatory process associated with scleritis may be caused by immune complex-related vascular damage (type III hypersensitivity) and subsequent chronic granulomatous response (type IV hypersensitivity).

Treatment is aimed at keeping the inflammatory response in check with high-dose systemic steroids. This goal is especially important in necrotizing scleritis. Additional treatment measures include pain medication, systemic anti-inflammatory agents, topical cyclosporine, and methotrexate. Some patients require scleral grafting. If left untreated, scleritis can progress to scleral thinning, scleral defects, anterior uveitis, keratitis, cataract, glaucoma, posterior uveitis, and visual loss.

Episcleritis

Episcleritis, an inflammation affecting the episcleral tissue between the conjunctiva and the sclera [50], produces a minimally painful red eye, with no visual symptoms (see Table 5). There are two types of episcleritis: simple and nodular. Most cases are idiopathic, but others are associated with collagen vascular disease such as rheumatoid arthritis, lupus erythematosus, or gout. The patient can be assured that this is a self-limiting disease. Anti-inflammatory agents can provide comfort.

Corneal ulcer

A corneal ulcer is a lesion that involves degradation of the corneal stroma. This condition is associated with inflammation, either sterile or infectious. It always begins with an epithelial defect that leads to stromal degradation, and corneal ulcers are painful. The anterior chamber should be examined closely for hypopyon (the presence of inflammatory exudates). The identification of an infectious or noninfectious cause will direct the clinical management (Table 6). Ulcers require immediate ophthalmologic consultation.

Contact-lens–induced peripheral ulceration (CLPU) is a common adverse response associated with wearing hydrogel lenses, especially on an extended-wear schedule [51,52]. Bacteriologic examination of lenses at the time of an event has demonstrated the presence of staphylococci species [53] and *Pseudomonas* organisms [51,52]. The suspected causal relationship between bacterial contamination and the development of contact-lens–induced ulcer is a controversial concept, but there is general agreement that contact lens wearers with peripheral corneal ulcer should be treated initially with topical antibiotics [54]. An eye with a CLPU or an abrasion should never be patched because a devastating *Pseudomonas* infection could develop.

Endophthalmitis

Endophthalmitis, typically a complication of cataract surgery, is a true ocular emergency. It develops several days after surgery, when the patient

Table 6
Causes of corneal ulcer

Infectious causes	Immune-related causes	Noninfectious causes
Bacterial (staphylococci, *Pseudomonas aeruginosa*, *Aeromonas hydrophila*, and *Serratia liquefaciens*)	Wegener's granulomatosis	Chemical burns
Fungal	Rheumatoid arthritis	Burns
Acanthamoeba	—	Sicca
Herpes simplex	—	Neurotrophic
Herpes zoster virus	—	Lid abnormalities caused by inadequate blink, facial palsy, proptosis, thyroid disease
Contact-lens–related	—	Contact-lens related; medicamentosa (drops); atopic; basement membrane; abnormalities; factitious

experiences a sudden onset of pain and reduction in vision. The patient will complain of seeing "floaters." The practitioner should identify a surgical incision on the cornea, a red eye with circumlimbal flush, anterior chamber cells, hypopyon, and posterior vitritis resulting in poor red reflex. A purulent discharge may be seen on the lid margin or eye lashes.

Endophthalmitis caused by *H influenzae* has been documented occurring from 6 days up to 18 months after invasive eye surgery. Treatment must be prompt and begun empirically because endophthalmitis can have a poor visual outcome if not treated aggressively [55].

An ophthalmologist should be consulted early in the evaluation. Emergency treatment should begin with class and dose of intravenous antibiotics. The majority of patients will require intravitreal injections, vitreous tap, subjunctival steroids, or vitrectomy to prevent a loss of the eye [56].

Acute vision loss

Cranial arteritis, giant cell arteritis, and temporal arteritis are the descriptive terms for a condition of adulthood (>50 years of age) that can lead to vision loss [57,58]. The patient complains of a headache and has severe visual complaints, malaise, myalgia, weight loss, and jaw claudication. The practitioner may find tenderness, redness, and swelling of the ipsilateral superficial temporal artery.

Classic abnormal laboratory findings include an erythrocyte sedimentation rate (ESR) of more than 100 min/h and an elevated level of C-reactive protein. Fundoscopic examination will demonstrate swelling of the optic nerve head. The inflammatory process has a tendency to affect the ophthalmic and the posterior ciliary arteries [58].

The practitioner must have a low threshold of suspicion to evaluate older individuals for this condition because irreversible visual loss can occur in up to 50% of untreated patients [57]. An early diagnosis and steroid therapy improve the chance of visual improvement [34]. This diagnosis should not be dismissed because the ESR is "not high enough" or the patient lacks "significant" arterial tenderness [58]. Treatment must be initiated at once with intravenous methylprednisolone at a dose of 20 mg to 100 mg. Patients may require treatment for 6 months to 2 years [57]. Consultation with an ophthalmologist and a neurologist is indicated.

Disorders of the lids and ocular soft tissues

Ultraviolet keratitis

Ultraviolet (UV) keratitis is an injury to the cornea caused by ultraviolet waves. The classic finding is the "starry night" pattern of fluorescein dye uptake. Symptoms are delayed for 8 to 12 hours after exposure to UV light, for example, from a welder's torch. Systemic analgesics are often required, and topical antibiotics typically are prescribed [59].

There are compelling reasons to counsel patients on the adverse effects of UV radiation and to offer them various protective options [5]. Sunglasses and UV-blocking ophthalmic lenses are the means of protection most commonly selected. The new UV-blocking hydrogel contact lenses are a recent addition to our armamentarium.

Snow blindness

The cornea can be injured within an hour of absorbing ultraviolet B rays. Snow blindness produces intense eye pain, blurred vision, and a diffuse punctate keratopathy. This condition is an indication for eye patching. Systemic analgesics are often required, and topical antibiotics typically are prescribed. Topical steroids can be prescribed if the cause does not include a bacterial or viral infection.

Pterygium and pinguecula

Pterygia arise from limbal epithelial cells [60]. They are fleshy appearing limbal lesions that appear to be creeping onto the cornea. An association between a pterygium formation and cataracts is suspected [61]. Recurrence is common.

Pingueculae are colored, raised growths that form on the conjunctiva. Whereas pterygia appear to be moving over the edge of the cornea, pingueculae appear to be nodules or bumps on the bulbar conjunctiva. Treatment requires that the patient be reassured. A borderline association between pinguecula and cataract formation has been reported [61].

The ultimate treatment, if any, for pterygia and pingueculae should occur in consultation with an ophthalmologist. However, the primary care provider can monitor the patient's symptoms and progression of these soft tissue conditions and serve as the patient's advocate for additional evaluation.

Hordeolum and chalazion

A hordeolum, commonly called a stye, is an acute, suppurative inflammation of the glands of Zeis and sweat glands or hair follicles, caused commonly by staphylococci infection. An external hordeolum points toward the skin surface, whereas an internal hordeolum erupts from the meibomian glands and points inwardly or externally [62]. A chalazion is an obstructed meibomian gland that produces swelling within the lid surface. The lid margin is normal.

The application of a warm compress and gentle massage can facilitate spontaneous resolution of hordeolum and chalazion. A topical antibiotic can be applied if the lesion causes eye irritation or local cellulitis. If cellulitis develops around a chalazion or if symptoms persist, surgical drainage may be required.

Dacryocystitis

Dacryocystitis appears as a painful, swollen, red, medially located mass that produces swelling and tenderness along the temporal aspect of the upper eyelid. *Staphylococcus aureus* is the most common offending organism. Several bacterial species have been associated with chronic dacryocystitis in adults [63], in whom gram-positive cocci are the predominant pathogens [64]. In adults, a bacterial cause is common, whereas in children, a viral cause is common. *H influenzae* should be considered as the causative agent in children who have not been vaccinated against that organism. Topical ophthalmic and systemic antibiotics are required for these conditions, and treatment can include applying cool compresses and prescribing oral antibiotics.

Cellulitis

Preseptal cellulitis can be caused by direct trauma, contiguous skin infections, or sinusitis. The practitioner must have a high index of suspicion for deep infections. Additional imaging studies such as ultrasonography, CT, and MRI frequently are required to reach an accurate diagnosis. Without prompt diagnosis and treatment, the infection can spread into the globe, causing endophthalmitis. Systemic antibiotics are required [65,66].

Orbital cellulitis also requires urgent treatment. The patient will present with unilateral proptosis, swelling with erythema of the eyelids, pain with extraocular movement, an afferent pupil defect, and decreased visual acuity. The cause can be a contiguous ethmoid sinus infection or a dental or soft tissue infection caused by *Staphylococcus* species, *H influenzae*, beta-hemolytic streptococcus, or *S pneumoniae* [66,67]. The incidence of *H influenza* infections has been waning since the advent of a vaccine against the organism [67].

The evaluation should include a CT scan of the sinuses and cranium. Treatment typically requires hospitalization, systemic antibiotics, and surgical drainage [65,66]. Left untreated, orbital cellulitis can progress to meningitis and cavernous sinus thrombosis.

Lens dislocation

Partial or complete lens dislocation, also known as ectopia lentis, may be caused by hereditary conditions, direct trauma, or homocystinemia [69]. Hereditary ectopia lentis usually is bilateral and associated with other congenital glaucoma, aniridia, or Ehlers–Danlos or Marfan's syndrome [68,69].

Ectopia lentis can cause various amounts of visual acuity loss, depending on the type and degree of dislocation and the presence of other ocular abnormalities [70]. The patient may complain of clear or blurry vision, depending on the position of the dislocated lens. A condition known as iridodonesis refers to a trembling of the lens with head movement. Iritis and glaucoma are complications of lens dislocation. Spontaneous ectopia lentis requires the combined evaluation and treatment efforts of the primary care provider and ophthalmologist because the cause must be determined (hereditary or metabolic), and the treatment must be tailored to the patient based on associated conditions [71]. In many cases, a dislocated lens is not treated [70].

Acute angle-closure glaucoma and elevated intraocular pressure

Impaired outflow of aqueous humor causes elevated intraocular pressure (IOP). In open-angle glaucoma, impaired outflow results from the dysfunction of the drainage system. In angle-closure glaucoma, impaired outflow results from the occlusion of the anterior chamber angle itself, impairing access of the aqueous to the drainage system [72]. Ocular hypertension can be precipitated by the administration of a mydriatic drug. Another common precipitating event is moving from daylight into a darkened environment, such as a movie theater. Regardless of the cause, ocular hypertension is defined as an IOP greater than 21 mm Hg [72].

Patients with angle-closure glaucoma have ocular and facial pain, unilateral blurring of vision, colored haloes around lights, nausea, and vomiting. Acuity will be reduced in the affected eye. The pupil will be fixed and mid-dilated. A deep conjunctival injection appears around the iris.

The practitioner has a large arsenal of topical medications that will quickly lower the IOP (Table 7), including β-blockers (eg, betaxolol, 0.125%; and timolol, 0.5%); carbonic anhydrase inhibitors (eg, dorzolamide, 2%; and brinzolamide, 1%); and prostaglandin F_{2a} analogs (eg, latanoprost, 0.005%; bimatoprost, 0.03%; and travoprost, 0.004%). One, two, or three such agents should be readily available in the primary care office. Medications such as timolol and dorzolamide can be administered concurrently [72–78]. In addition to topical agents, oral acetazolamide (500 mg) can be administered if the IOP is not lowered fast enough, as tested by tonometry, which should be performed frequently during the emergency therapeutic course.

Table 7
Examples of ophthalmic medications

Example	Bottletop color	Action
Tropicamide	Red	Pupil dilation (mydriasis)
Pilocarpine	Green	Pupil constriction (miosis)
Timolol maleate[a]	Yellow	Decrease aqueous humor production
Timolol XL[a]	Yellow	Decrease aqueous humor production
Betaxolol[a]	Yellow	Decrease aqueous humor production
Tetracaine	White	Anesthetic
Lacrilube	Blue	Lubricants and irrigating solutions

[a] **Caution:** these medications may produce systemic side effects.

Herpes simplex keratitis

Herpes simplex keratitis produces localized pain and a foreign body sensation. Fluorescein stain demonstrates a dendritic pattern. Treatment includes antiviral agents (systemic and topical) and a cycloplegic agent.

Herpes zoster conjunctivitis

Herpes zoster is uniformly a uniocular lesion involving the fifth cranial nerve. The cornea may be involved alone or along with a branch of the nasociliary nerve, which supplies the tip of nose and the cornea. If the tip of nose is involved (Hutchinson's sign), corneal involvement should be suspected. Ocular tearing, irritation, typical skin lesions, and photophobia are additional features of herpes zoster conjunctivitis.

Treatment includes oral acyclovir. Topical antiviral agents typically are not beneficial. Adjunctive treatment should include the application of a topical lubricant, prescribing a systemic analgesic, and treating other zoster complications.

Eclipse burn

Eclipse burn, or sungazer's retinopathy, is the severe photocoagulation of the macula. Central vision is lost, producing a "gun barrel" central visual field defect. The remaining visual acuity may be 20/200 or worse.

Hysterical and functional blindness

Hysterical blindness, functional vision loss, and psychogenic amaurosis [79] are terms used to describe the experience of blindness without ocular or cerebral disease. Hysterical blindness can be a feature of hysterical conversion reaction in children [80]. Functional blindness (not to be confused with functional visual impairment) can be caused by benign essential blepharospasm (ie, involuntary, uncontrollable eyelid closure or segmental dystonia, that is, movement disorders involving the lower face and neck) [81]. These disorders typically present in the fifth and sixth decades of life. Essential blepharospasm is particularly debilitating because the involuntary eyelid closure may result in functional blindness despite an otherwise normal visual pathway. Definitive treatment of hysterical and functional blindness requires a collaborative diagnostic effort by an ophthalmologist, a mental health expert, and the primary care provider.

Hyphema

Hyphema is the condition of having blood in the clear aqueous fluid in the anterior chamber. The presence of even the slightest amount of blood causes some degree of decreased vision. The patient may complain of pain caused by elevated IOP. It is important to examine the patient for associated orbital and globe trauma, particularly penetrating trauma, lens injury, and posterior chamber injury.

Treatment is based on the cause and severity of the hyphema. Frequently, the blood is resorbed over a period of days to weeks. IOP can be measured if the globe and cornea are intact. Patients with significant hyphema must rest and avoid strenuous activity to allow the blood to disperse. Bleeding worse than the original episode recurs during the first 5 days after injury in 2% of blue-eyed individuals and in 40% of African Americans.

A grading system commonly used to describe hyphema is based on the amount of blood in the anterior chamber (Table 8) [82]. The grade correlates positively with the IOP and the amount of blood that has been resorbed. Spontaneous, atraumatic bleeding in the eye should prompt an investigation for the use of anticoagulant medication or the presence of sickle cell anemia, hemophilia, or von Willebrand's disease (vascular hemophilia). Sickle cell trait alone is a risk factor for rebleeding, elevated IOP, and visual impairment in children who have traumatic hyphemas [83].

The factors to consider when deciding the course of treatment for a patient with hyphema (whether to treat, admit the patient to a hospital, follow the patient in his or her home, or refer the patient to an ophthalmologist) include the cause and grade of the hyphema, the IOP level, and the patient's overall safety, considering the degree of visual impairment. In consultation with an ophthalmologist, the primary care physician can decide on the use of a topical cycloplegic agent, corticosteroids, or aminocaproic acid. The patient should be instructed to refrain from activity and wear a rigid eye shield during activity. Mixed results have been reported concerning the use of topical aminocaproic acid gel. Rebleeding rates, clot resorption time, and the effect on IOP must be monitored closely with this therapy [84,85]. The primary care physician must coordinate this treatment approach with an ophthalmologist, who will assist in evaluating the patient.

Table 8
Grading system for hyphema based on amount of blood in the anterior chamber

Grade	Criteria
1	Less than one-forth of the visible volume of the anterior chamber
2	One-forth to one-half of the visible volume of the anterior chamber
3	One-half to three-forths of the visible volume of the anterior chamber
4	Complete filling of the visible anterior chamber[a]

[a] An "eight-ball hemorrhage" refers to an anterior chamber completely filled with black clots.

Adapted from Sowka JW, Gurwood AS, Kabat AG. Hyphema. In: Handbook of Ocular Disease Management. Jobson Publishing LLC, 2000–2001. Available at: http://www.revoptom.com/handbook/sect4f.htm. Accessed on July 8, 2005.

Selected traumatic eye disorders

Corneal abrasions

In a patient who presents with a corneal abrasion, fluorescein stain pools in the corneal defect. The "ice rink sign" refers to multiple vertical abrasions that resemble the marks left on ice by skate blades. The lid must be inverted and inspected for a foreign body. Treatment consists of a topical antibiotic, an oral analgesic, and a short-acting cycloplegic. Patching is generally unnecessary. As mentioned previously, contact-lens–induced corneal injuries should never be patched.

Globe perforation

Globe perforation should be suspected in a patient who presents with a penetrating wound of the lid or with a vitreous hemorrhage. Ocular rupture can be diagnosed if a stream of clear fluid dilutes topically applied fluorescein (Seidel test). Globe perforations should be protected with a firm shield that does not touch the globe, and urgent referral to an ophthalmologist is essential. Commercially available shields or a shield constructed from the bottom half of a paper cup offers suitable eye protection. Tetanus immunization or vaccination should be administered if needed, as well as a systemic antibiotic.

References

[1] Xiang H, Stallones L, Chen G, et al. Work-related eye injuries treated in hospital emergency departments in the US. Am J Ind Med 2005;48(1):57–62.
[2] Rahmani B, Tielsch JM, Katz J, et al. The cause-specific prevalence of visual impairment in an urban population: the Baltimore Eye Survey. Ophthalmology 1996;103(11):1721–6.
[3] Ramrattan RS, Wolfs RC, Panda-Jonas S, et al. Prevalence and causes of visual field loss in the elderly and associations with impairment in daily functioning: the Rotterdam Study. Arch Ophthalmol 2001;119(12):1788–94.
[4] Kaiserman I, Kaiserman N, Nakar S, et al. The effect of combination pharmacotherapy on the prescription trends of glaucoma medications. J Glaucoma 2005;14(2):157–60.
[5] Bergmanson JP, Sheldon TM. Ultraviolet radiation revisited. CLAO J 1997;23(3):196–204.
[6] Brown GC, Magargal LE, Shields JA, et al. Retinal arterial obstruction in children and young adults. Ophthalmology 1981;88(1):18–25.
[7] Hayreh SS, Zimmerman MB, Kimura A, et al. Central retinal artery occlusion: retinal survival time. Exp Eye Res 2004;78(3):723–36.
[8] Rumelt S, Brown GC. Update on treatment of retinal arterial occlusions. Curr Opin Ophthalmol 2003;14(3):139–41.
[9] Durukan AH, Akar Y, Bayraktar MZ, et al. Combined retinal artery and vein occlusion in a patient with systemic lupus erythematosus and antiphospholipid syndrome. Can J Ophthalmol 2005;40(1):87–9.
[10] Au A, O'Day J. Review of severe vaso-occlusive retinopathy in systemic lupus erythematosus and the antiphospholipid syndrome: associations, visual outcomes, complications and treatment. Clin Experiment Ophthalmol 2004;32(1):87–100.

[11] Salvarani C, Cimino L, Macchioni P, et al. Risk factors for visual loss in an Italian population-based cohort of patients with giant cell arteritis. Arthritis Rheum 2005;53(2):293–7.
[12] Galasso JM, Jay WM. An occult case of giant cell arteritis presenting with combined anterior ischemic optic neuropathy and cilioretinal artery occlusion. Semin Ophthalmol 2004; 19(3–4):75–7.
[13] Chan WM, Liu DT, Lam DS. Images in haematology: combined central retinal artery and vein occlusions as the presenting signs of ocular relapse in acute lymphoblastic leukaemia. Br J Haematol 2005;128(2):134.
[14] Schneider U, Hermann A, Ernemann U, et al. Central retinal artery occlusion secondary to spontaneous internal carotid artery dissection. Retina 2004;24(6):979–81.
[15] Susac JO, Calabrese LH, Baylin E, et al. Branch retinal artery occlusions as the presenting feature of primary central nervous system vasculitis. Clin Exp Rheumatol 2004; 22(Suppl 36):S70–4.
[16] Ozdek S, Yulek F, Gurelik G, et al. Simultaneous central retinal vein and retinal artery branch occlusions in two patients with homocystinaemia. Eye 2004;18(9):942–5.
[17] Nakagawa T, Hirata A, Inoue N, et al. A case of bilateral central retinal artery obstruction with patent foramen ovale. Acta Ophthalmol Scand 2004;82(1):111–2.
[18] Foroozan R. Combined central retinal artery and vein occlusion from orbital inflammatory pseudotumour. Clin Experiment Ophthalmol 2004;32(4):435–7.
[19] Sanchez-Tocino H, Garcia-Layana A, Salinas-Alaman A, et al. Central retinal vascular occlusion by orbital pseudotumor. Retina 2004;24(3):455–8.
[20] Imai E, Kunikata H, Udono T, et al. Branch retinal artery occlusion: a complication of iron-deficiency anemia in a young adult with a rectal carcinoid. Tohoku J Exp Med 2004;203(2):141–4.
[21] Shukla D, Mohan KC, Rao N, et al. Posterior scleritis causing combined central retinal artery and vein occlusion. Retina 2004;24(3):467–9.
[22] Sawada T, Harino S, Ikeda T. Central retinal artery occlusion in a patient with fibromuscular dysplasia. Retina 2004;24(3):461–4.
[23] Costello F, Gilberg S, Karsh J, et al. Bilateral simultaneous central retinal artery occlusions in Wegener granulomatosis. J Neuroophthalmol 2005;25(1):29–32.
[24] Peng YJ, Fang PC, Huang WT. Central retinal artery occlusion in Wegener's granulomatosis: a case report and review of the literature. Can J Ophthalmol 2004;39(7):785–9.
[25] Umeed S, Shafquat S. Commotio-retinae and central retinal artery occlusion after blunt ocular trauma. Eye 2004;18(3):333–4.
[26] Kymionis GD, Tsilimbaris MK, Christodoulakis EB, et al. Late onset branch retinal artery occlusion following coronary angiography. Acta Ophthalmol Scand 2005;83(1):122–3.
[27] Zein WM, Hadi UM, Bashshur ZF, et al. Branch retinal artery occlusion following embolization of a maxillary sinus tumor. J Med Liban 2003;51(4):228–30.
[28] Smith WK, Nixon I, Pfleiderer AG. Central retinal artery occlusion following a total laryngectomy. J Otolaryngol 2004;33(2):130–2.
[29] Halfon MJ, Bonardo P, Valiensi S, et al. Central retinal artery occlusion and ophthalmoplegia following spinal surgery. Br J Ophthalmol 2004;88(10):1350–2.
[30] Vinerovsky A, Rath EZ, Rehany U, et al. Central retinal artery occlusion after peribulbar anesthesia. J Cataract Refract Surg 2004;30(4):913–5.
[31] Kondamudi V, Reddy R, Kondamudi N, et al. Sudden painless unilateral vision loss caused by branch retinal artery occlusion: implications for the primary care physician. Am J Med Sci 2004;327(1):44–6.
[32] Hayreh SS, Kolder HE, Weingeist TA. Central retinal artery occlusion and retinal tolerance time. Ophthalmology 1980;87(1):75–8.
[33] Mueller AJ, Neubauer AS, Schaller U, et al, for the European Assessment Group for Lysis in the Eye. Evaluation of minimally invasive therapies and rationale for a prospective randomized trial to evaluate selective intra-arterial lysis for clinically complete central retinal artery occlusion. Arch Ophthalmol 2003;121(10):1377–81.

[34] Hayreh SS, Zimmerman B, Kardon RH. Visual improvement with corticosteroid therapy in giant cell arteritis: report of a large study and review of literature. Acta Ophthalmol Scand 2002;80(4):355–67.
[35] Wray SH. The management of acute visual failure. J Neurol Neurosurg Psychiatry 1993; 56(3):234–40.
[36] Beiran I, Goldenberg I, Adir Y, et al. Early hyperbaric oxygen therapy for retinal artery occlusion. Eur J Ophthalmol 2001;11(4):345–50.
[37] Nilsson P, Larsson EM, Maly-Sundgren P, et al. Predicting the outcome of optic neuritis evaluation of risk factors after 30 years of follow-up. J Neurol 2005;252(4):396–402.
[38] Liu JZ, Brown P, Tselis A. Unilateral retrobulbar optic neuritis due to varicella zoster virus in a patient with AIDS: a case report and review of the literature. J Neurol Sci 2005; 237(1–2):97–101.
[39] Rozenbaum D, Baruchin AM, Dafna Z. Chemical burns of the eye with special reference to alkali burns. Burns 1991;17(2):136–40.
[40] Davis AR, Ali QK, Aclimandos WA, et al. Topical steroid use in the treatment of ocular alkali burns. Br J Ophthalmol 1997;81:732–4.
[41] Brodovsky SC, McCarty CA, Snibson G, et al. Management of alkali burns: an 11-year retrospective review. Ophthalmology 2000;107(10):1829–35.
[42] Soderberg K, Kuusinen P, Mathieu L, et al. An improved method for emergent decontamination of ocular and dermal hydrofluoric acid splashes. Vet Hum Toxicol 2004;46(4):216–8.
[43] McCulley JP. Ocular hydrofluoric acid burns: animal model, mechanism of injury and therapy. Trans Am Ophthalmol Soc 1990;88:649–84.
[44] Beiran I, Miller B, Bentur Y. The efficacy of calcium gluconate in ocular hydrofluoric acid burns. Hum Exp Toxicol 1997;16(4):223–8.
[45] Ullman S, Roussel TJ, Culbertson WW, et al. *Neisseria gonorrhoeae* keratoconjunctivitis. Ophthalmology 1987;94(5):525–31.
[46] Pareek SS. Conjunctivitis caused by beta-lactamase-producing *Neisseria gonorrhoeae*. Sex Transm Dis 1985;12(3):159–60.
[47] Kestelyn P, Bogaerts J, Stevens AM, et al. Treatment of adult gonococcal keratoconjunctivitis with oral norfloxacin. Am J Ophthalmol 1989;108(5):516–23.
[48] Ruppert SD. Differential diagnosis of pediatric conjunctivitis (red eye). Nurse Pract 1996; 21(7):12–24.
[49] Maza MS. Scleritis. [eMedicine.com Web site]. June 10, 2005. Available at: http://www.emedicine.com/oph/topic642.htm. Accessed July 15, 2005.
[50] Roy Sr H. Episcleritis. [eMedicine.com Web site]. December 10, 2004. Available at: http://www.emedicine.com/oph/topic641.htm. Accessed July 15, 2005.
[51] Venkata N, Sharma S, Gora R, et al. Clinical presentation of microbial keratitis with daily wear frequent-replacement hydrogel lenses: a case series. CLAO J 2002;28(3):165–8.
[52] Sankaridurg PR, Vuppala N, Sreedharan A, et al. Gram negative bacteria and contact lens induced acute red eye. Indian J Ophthalmol 1996;44(1):29–32.
[53] Wu P, Stapleton F, Willcox MD. The causes of and cures for contact lens-induced peripheral ulcer. Eye Contact Lens 2003;29(Suppl 1):S63–6 [discussion: S83–4, S192–4].
[54] Donshik PC, Suchecki JK, Ehlers WH. Peripheral corneal infiltrates associated with contact lens wear. Trans Am Ophthalmol Soc 1995;93:49–60 [discussion: 60–4].
[55] Yoder DM, Scott IU, Flynn HW Jr, et al. Endophthalmitis caused by *Haemophilus influenzae*. Ophthalmology 2004;111(11):2023–6.
[56] Chaudhry NA, Lavaque AJ, Scott IU, et al. A cluster of patients with acute-onset endophthalmitis following cataract surgery. Ophthalmic Surg Lasers Imaging 2005;36(3): 205–10.
[57] Spiera R, Spiera H. Inflammatory disease in older adults: cranial arteritis. Geriatrics 2004; 59(12):25–9.
[58] Gurwood AS, Brilliant R, Malloy KA. The enigma of giant cell arteritis: multidisciplinary management of two cases. J Am Optom Assoc 1998;69(8):501–9.

[59] Stokkermans TJ, Dunbar MT. Solar retinopathy in a hospital-based primary care clinic. J Am Optom Assoc 1998;69(10):625–36.
[60] Gebhardt M, Mentlein R, Schaudig U, et al. Differential expression of vascular endothelial growth factor implies the limbal origin of pterygia. Ophthalmology 2005;112(6):1023–30.
[61] Pham TQ, Wang JJ, Rochtchina E, et al. Pterygium, pinguecula, and 5-year incidence of cataract. Am J Ophthalmol 2005;139(6):1126–8.
[62] Kiratli HK, Akar Y. Multiple recurrent hordeola associated with selective IgM deficiency. J AAPOS 2001;5(1):60–1.
[63] Chaudhry IA, Shamsi FA, Al-Rashed W. Bacteriology of chronic dacryocystitis in a tertiary eye care center. Ophthal Plast Reconstr Surg 2005;21(3):207–10.
[64] Sun X, Liang Q, Luo S, et al. Microbiological analysis of chronic dacryocystitis. Ophthalmic Physiol Opt 2005;25(3):261–3.
[65] Howe L, Jones NS. Guidelines for the management of periorbital cellulitis/abscess. Clin Otolaryngol 2004;29(6):725–8.
[66] Weiss A, Friendly D, Eglin K, et al. Bacterial periorbital and orbital cellulitis in childhood. Ophthalmology 1983;90(3):195–203.
[67] Ambati BK, Ambati J, Azar N, et al. Periorbital and orbital cellulitis before and after the advent of *Haemophilus influenzae* type B vaccination. Ophthalmology 2000;107(8):1450–3.
[68] Young TL. Ophthalmic genetics/inherited eye disease. Curr Opin Ophthalmol 2003;14(5): 296–303.
[69] Peter NM, Nath R, Tranos PG, et al. Bilateral lens subluxation associated with atopic eczema. Eur J Ophthalmol 2005;15(3):409–11.
[70] Nelson LB, Maumenee IH. Ectopia lentis. Surv Ophthalmol 1982;27(3):143–60.
[71] Cross HE. Differential diagnosis and treatment of dislocated lenses. Birth Defects Orig Artic Ser 1976;12(3):335–46.
[72] Distelhorst JS, Hughes GM. Open-angle glaucoma. Am Fam Physician 2003;67(9):1937–44.
[73] Michaud JE, Friren B, for the International Brinzolamide Adjunctive Study Group. Comparison of topical brinzolamide 1% and dorzolamide 2% eye drops given twice daily in addition to timolol 0.5% in patients with primary open-angle glaucoma or ocular hypertension. Am J Ophthalmol 2001;132(2):235–43.
[74] Strahlman E, Tipping R. Vogel R for the International Dorzolamide Study Group. A double-masked, randomized 1-year study comparing dorzolamide (Trusopt), timolol, and betaxolol. Arch Ophthalmol 1995;113(8):1009–16.
[75] Silver LH, for the Brinzolamide Primary Therapy Study Group. Clinical efficacy and safety of brinzolamide (Azopt), a new topical carbonic anhydrase inhibitor for primary open-angle glaucoma and ocular hypertension. Am J Ophthalmol 1998;126(3):400–8.
[76] Toor A, Chanis RA, Polikoff LA, Fahim MM, et al. Additivity of pilocarpine to bimatoprost in ocular hypertension and early glaucoma. J Glaucoma 2005;14(3):243–8.
[77] Parrish RK, Palmberg P, Sheu WP, for the XLT Study Group. A comparison of latanoprost, bimatoprost, and travoprost in patients with elevated intraocular pressure: a 12-week, randomized, masked-evaluator multicenter study. Am J Ophthalmol 2003;135(5):688–703.
[78] Brandt JD, VanDenburgh AM, Chen K, et al, for the Bimatoprost Study Group. Comparison of once- or twice-daily bimatoprost with twice-daily timolol in patients with elevated IOP: a 3-month clinical trial. Ophthalmology 2001;108(6):1023–32.
[79] Ziegler DK, Schlemmer RB. Familial psychogenic blindness and headache: a case study. J Clin Psychiatry 1994;55(3):114–7.
[80] Bangash IH, Worley G, Kandt RS. Hysterical conversion reactions mimicking neurological disease. Am J Dis Child 1988;142(11):1203–6.
[81] Holds JB, White GL Jr, Thiese SM, et al. Facial dystonia, essential blepharospasm and hemifacial spasm. Am Fam Physician 1991;43(6):2113–20.
[82] Sowka JW, Gurwood AS, Kabat AG. Hyphema. In: Handbook of ocular disease management. Jobson Publishing, LLC. 2000-2001. Available at: http://www.revoptom.com/handbook/sect4f.htm. Accessed July 8, 2005.

[83] Nasrullah A, Kerr NC. Sickle cell trait as a risk factor for secondary hemorrhage in children with traumatic hyphema. Am J Ophthalmol 1997;123(6):783–90.
[84] Pieramici DJ, Goldberg MF, Melia M, et al. A phase III, multicenter, randomized, placebo-controlled clinical trial of topical aminocaproic acid (Caprogel) in the management of traumatic hyphema. Ophthalmology 2003;110(11):2106–12.
[85] Karkhaneh R, Naeeni M, Chams H, et al. Topical aminocaproic acid to prevent rebleeding in cases of traumatic hyphema. Eur J Ophthalmol 2003;13(1):57–61.

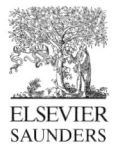

Otolaryngologic Emergencies in the Outpatient Setting

Walter G. Belleza, MD*, Suzanne Kalman, MD

Division of Emergency Medicine, University of Maryland School of Medicine, Baltimore, MD, USA

Primary care clinicians encounter otolaryngologic conditions on a daily basis. Many of the more common conditions, such as pharyngitis, sinusitis, otitis media, and otitis externa, are self-limited and resolve without requiring extensive treatment or evaluation by a subspecialist. Other conditions, such as trauma and epistaxis, receive an evaluation in an emergency department or are self-treated at home by the patient. As result of improvements in general medical care and antimicrobial therapy, the number of complications from the aforementioned conditions has declined significantly.

Unfortunately, the decline also has led to a lack of familiarity with the pathophysiology, clinical presentation, and treatment of many potentially life-threatening conditions. As a result, patients may present with subtle signs of serious conditions that may go unappreciated if the clinician is not diligent. The presentation may also be obscured by the concomitant use of antibiotics, pain medication, or the presence of a pre-existing disease states such as diabetes. The subtlety of many clinical findings and the relative rarity of complications such as deep tissue infections, intracranial complications, and vascular thrombosis can lead to a misdiagnosis and result in significant delays in evaluation, referral, and treatment. Additionally, the location of these complications and their close proximity to neurologic, cardiovascular, and airway structures can result in rapid, severe compromise if not diagnosed appropriately.

The incidence of complications such as deep tissue infections and intracranial complications is rare compared with other medical conditions. Complications such as brain abscesses account for only 1 per 10,000 hospital admissions in some studies [1]. Unfortunately, many of these

---

* Corresponding author. Division of Emergency Medicine, University of Maryland School of Medicine, 110 South Paca Street, 6th Floor, Suite 200, Baltimore, MD 21201.

0025-7125/06/$ - see front matter © 2006 Elsevier Inc. All rights reserved.
doi:10.1016/j.mcna.2005.12.001 *medical.theclinics.com*

complications will afflict those who are most susceptible to significant sequelae but are the least likely to seek immediate medical care, including immigrants, the impoverished, alcoholics, the elderly, and the immunocompromised. Although most of these patients who experience severe distress or hemodynamic instability from complications will present to any emergency department or subspecialist, some patients may present initially to primary care physicians.

This article familiarizes the clinician with the pathophysiology and clinical presentation of potentially serious otolaryngologic conditions that may be encountered in the outpatient setting, including suppurative complications of sinusitis, otitis media and externa, and infections involving the oropharynx. Other conditions such as trauma, hemorrhage, foreign bodies, and complications related to piercing of the ear and tongue are also discussed. Because these conditions can potentially produce life-threatening complications, most of the conditions discussed will require definitive diagnoses and treatment within an inpatient setting.

Complications of sinusitis

Nearly 20 million cases of bacterial sinusitis occur in the United States every year [2]. Because of aggressive antibiotic therapy and the natural course of the disease, the majority of these cases resolve without significant sequelae. Life-threatening complications result from bacterial extension into the orbital and intracranial spaces, through direct invasion or from septic thrombophlebitis. These complications can be subdivided into those involving the orbit, intracranial spaces, and vascular sinuses.

Orbital complications

Complications involving the orbit generally can be subdivided into those that occur anterior and posterior to the orbital septum. The orbital septum is formed from a continuation of the periosteum of the superior and inferior orbital margins, which merge into the palpebral fascia of both eyelids. Infections that occur anterior to the orbital septum usually are uncomplicated, whereas those that occur posterior to the septum may lead to a variety of complications. An anatomic classification of inflammatory processes involving the orbit was first described by Smith and Spencer [3] in 1948 and later revised by Chandler and colleagues (Table 1) [4].

The challenge facing both the primary care physician and specialist is to determine the degree of inflammatory involvement that exists in the patient who presents with a swollen orbit. In addition to infection, the clinician should also consider uveitis, dacryocystitis, trauma, contact allergy, neoplasm, or insect bites as the source of a swollen orbit.

The examination should focus on the appearance of the patient's globe, visual acuity, oculomotor ability, and the patient's overall clinical status.

Table 1
Chandler classification of orbital inflammation

Stage	Inflammation
I	Inflammatory edema
II	Orbital cellulitis
III	Subperiosteal abscess
IV	Orbital abscess
V	Cavernous sinus thrombosis

If the patient's visual acuity and oculomotor status cannot be assessed adequately, the patient should be referred immediately to an ophthalmologic specialist or an emergency department. Definitive treatment requires aggressive intravenous antibiotic therapy and surgical intervention. The only patient with a swollen orbit who could be sent home is one without vision loss, with upper eyelid edema alone, and in whom one can assure medical compliance and adequate follow-up care.

Periorbital cellulitis

Periorbital or preseptal cellulitis (Chandler stage I) is defined as an inflammation limited to the tissues of the eyelid. Sources of infection include sinusitis, trauma, insect bites, conjunctivitis, and upper respiratory infection [5]. The most common organisms include *Streptococcus pneumoniae, Staphylococcus aureus,* anaerobes, and coagulase-negative staphylococci.

Common clinical findings include unilateral periorbital erythema, edema, pain, and fever. The presence of other findings such as proptosis, diplopia, and visual loss should alert the physician to the presence of intraorbital involvement. Patients who have periorbital cellulitis usually are treated on an outpatient basis with broad-spectrum antibiotics and rarely develop complications.

Orbital complications

The maxillary and ethmoid sinuses form an integral component of the orbital structure, and infections in these areas are a significant cause of both periorbital cellulitis and orbital complications [6,7]. Other causes of orbital cellulitis include dacryocystitis and foreign bodies. Orbital involvement (Chandler stages II–V) represents a true emergency that may lead to complications such as meningitis, vision loss, cavernous sinus thrombosis, and frontal abscess.

Nearly all patients with intraorbital infection will have fever, soft tissue swelling, and pain, but the presence of orbital dysfunction will distinguish it from periorbital cellulitis. The orbital symptoms are caused primarily by either direct irritation of neural structures or the increase in intraorbital pressure produced by inflammation or infectious material. Symptoms include proptosis, chemosis, restriction of ocular movement, and visual disturbance if the process involves the orbital apex. The clinical symptoms of stages II through IV are similar, and the presence of a subperiosteal and orbital abscess is difficult to distinguish without the aid of a CT scan.

All patients who are suspected of having orbital cellulitis require admission to a facility with both ophthalmologic and otolaryngologic capabilities for definitive diagnosis and treatment. The diagnosis requires a CT scan, which can define the extent of orbital and periorbital involvement and visualize the sinuses. The most common pathogens are *Strep milleri, Strep pyogenes, Strep pneumoniae, Staph aureus*, and anaerobes if chronic sinusitis exists. Therefore, initial antibiotic therapy should include a broad-spectrum cephalosporin combined with an agent such as metronidazole. Further treatment is tailored on a case-by-case basis and may entail surgical or endoscopic drainage of the infection.

Frontal osteomyelitis: Pott's puffy tumor

Another complication of sinusitis is osteomyelitis of the frontal bone. Commonly known as Pott's puffy tumor, osteomyelitis of the frontal bone usually occurs secondary to frontal sinusitis and may occur in association with intracranial complications.

Infectious invasion of marrow can occur through contiguous invasion or through septic thrombophlebitic spread. Although it is secondary to frontal sinusitis, the most common causative agents are *Staph aureus* and anaerobes [8]. Patients usually will present with headache and a well-circumscribed swelling of the forehead that has progressively developed over several weeks to months. Because of its progressive nature, patients with frontal osteomyelitis should not present in extremis, unless an associated condition exists. The diagnosis is established by CT or MRI. Treatment involves the drainage of any abscess and the debridement of any infected bone.

Cavernous sinus thrombosis

If cavernous sinus thrombosis (Chandler stage V) is present, the patient will present with bilateral proptosis, opthalmoplegia, severe headache, sensory dysfunction, and visual loss. The headache usually is unilateral and retro-orbital, interferes with sleep, and is not relieved by analgesic medication. The opthalmoplegia may be external (caused by dysfunction of cranial nerves III, IV, and VI) or internal (caused by paralysis of the ciliary and iris apparatus). Sensory dysfunction may present as hypoesthesia or hyperesthesia of the area innervated by the first division of the trigeminal nerve. These symptoms usually develop acutely and within 1 week from the onset of the infectious process [9].

The physical examination reveals a febrile, toxic patient with periorbital edema, headaches, cranial nerve dysfunction, and papilledema. Classically, the periorbital edema is bilateral but may begin unilaterally and usually develops within 24 to 48 hours of the initial presentation [10]. The ocular examination should focus on extraocular muscle function, which may indicate dysfunction of cranial nerves III, IV, and VI. Pupillary examination may reveal either a dilated or small, unresponsive pupil that indicates dysfunction of the parasympathetic or sympathetic fibers of cranial nerve III, respectively. Papilledema and venous engorgement are late findings. If an extension develops into brain parenchyma or other vascular sinuses, dysphagia, seizures, hemiplegia, or obtundation may develop.

A definitive diagnosis requires either high-resolution CT scanning with 3-mm slice thicknesses or MR angiography that reveals an absence of flow through the venous system [11]. The primary goal of treatment is to eradicate the precipitating source of infection with aggressive intravenous antibiotic therapy.

Intracranial complications of sinusitis

Because of their anatomic location and venous drainage, sinus infections can lead to suppurative intracranial complications. These include, in order of increasing frequency, cavernous sinus thrombosis, meningitis, extradural abscess, intracranial abscess, and subdural empyema [12]. Currently, sinusitis is the source of 18% of brain abscesses, but it accounted for nearly 32% of brain abscesses in the preantibiotic era [13]. The sources most commonly implicated are the frontal, ethmoid, and sphenoid sinuses [14].

Infection can spread from the sinuses directly through anatomic and traumatic structural defects or by retrograde thrombophlebitis through the diploic or communicating veins. Contiguous suppuration is responsible for the majority of abscesses, whereas vascular channels are the primary means in subdural empyema. The most commonly cultured organisms include *Staph aureus*, *Streptococcus* species, *Haemophilus influenzae*, and *Bacteroides* species.

The most common clinical symptoms of sinusitis-induced intracranial complications are purulent rhinorrhea, fever, and a frontal or retro-orbital headache. Unfortunately, the similarity of symptoms with sinusitis itself may make it difficult to distinguish initially. The clinician should maintain a high level of vigilance for symptoms such as personality change or lethargy that may indicate the presence of an intracranial process.

This initial paucity of findings occurs more commonly in intracerebral abscesses, in which abscess formation begins slowly as an area of cerebritis that eventually coalesces into a focal lesion. Because abscess formation occurs in a neurologically quiescent area, the patient will not manifest symptoms until an abscess has grown large enough to cause either increased intracranial pressure or rupture. The time course of the disease process from symptom onset to presentation can range from hours to 1 month.

The classic clinical manifestations of brain abscesses are headache, fever, and focal neurologic deficits [15]. Other symptoms include seizures, nausea and vomiting, nuchal rigidity, and photophobia. Unfortunately, the classic triad of symptoms is present in less than 50% of patients [15].

A subdural empyema will present with more dramatic findings, such as systemic toxicity, nuchal rigidity, photophobia, cranial nerve deficits, seizures, and encephalopathy. Unlike brain abscesses, headaches are an uncommon complaint. The presence of these symptoms is a poor prognostic sign and an indication of a high mortality rate.

The definitive diagnostic test for intracranial complications is a MRI scan with gadolinium. Patients must be admitted to an intensive care unit at a facility with neurosurgical and otolaryngologic surgical capability. Treatment is tailored on a case-by-case basis, with patients receiving broad-spectrum antibiotic therapy that may be accompanied by surgical evacuation of the infected sinus and the intracranial process.

Complicated ear infections

Otitis media and otitis externa are common infections. Nearly 10% of adults will develop an external ear infection during their lifetime, whereas otitis media is the most common condition requiring antibiotic therapy in children [16,17]. Most infections are treated easily, but the anatomic structures of the internal and external ear allow infections to spread intracranially or into local bony structures. Once established, infections may spread further into the mastoid (Bezold's abscess), lower neck, or into vascular structures.

Malignant otitis externa

The anatomic structure of the external ear canal allows for the easy spread of an infectious process. The anterior cartilaginous portion of the canal contains the fissures of Santorini, which are embryonic channels through which neurovascular tissue passes. The inner osseous portion of the external ear canal contains little subcutaneous tissue, with the dermis in nearly direct contact with the periosteum. As a result, infection may occur through direct extension or vascular spread.

Malignant otitis externa (MOE) is an invasive infectious process that involves the temporal bone and its adjoining structures. It is primarily a complication of otitis externa and usually afflicts immunocompromised patients, such as diabetics, the elderly, the malnourished, and those with an underlying malignancy. It is believed that a preexisting depression of local defense mechanisms in the immunocompromised patient is a significant factor in the progression of malignant otitis externa.

The primary infectious agent is *Pseudomonas aeruginosa*, which can be introduced into the external canal from swimming pool water or inadvertent trauma (eg, cotton swabs). Once established, the infection spreads to the cartilaginous skeleton of the ear canal and eventually into the temporal bone where an osteitis develops. If it is left unchecked, the infection may spread into the base of the skull or into the cranium, resulting in extra-auricular symptoms.

The most common clinical complaint in MOE is severe, unremitting otalgia, which is present in nearly all patients [18]. Although discomfort is present in otitis externa, the severity of pain and its presence at night are distinguishing features [19]. Another significant symptom is purulent otorrhea, which may actually decrease as the disease progresses. As the infection spreads, it may result in extra-auricular symptoms such as trismus, cervical adenopathy, and cranial nerve palsies. The presence of a cranial nerve dysfunction indicates a poor prognosis [19].

The diagnosis of MOE first requires a high index of suspicion. MOE should be suspected in any diabetic or immunocompromised patient who presents with persistent external otitis and whose pain is worse at night. The physical examination usually reveals edema and erythema of the ear canal, along with the presence of granulation tissue in the external canal.

A CT scan is the diagnostic modality of choice and should be used to evaluate for the presence of intracranial complications. Treatment usually requires the use of a broad-spectrum antibiotic with antipseudomonal activity for 4 to 8 weeks.

Intracranial complications

As with sinusitis, the proximity of the inner ear to the cranium can result in a number of intracranial complications that may occur simultaneously, including meningitis, epidural and brain abscesses, lateral sinus thrombosis, and petrositis. The overall incidence of intracranial complications is less than 2%, and the most common complications are meningitis and brain abscesses [20,21]. The incidence of brain abscesses is relatively rare, with an incidence of 2 in 10,000 hospital visits [22]. The most commonly affected areas of the brain are the middle part of the temporal lobe and the lateral lobe of the cerebellum. Pathogens include *Proteus mirabilis, Enterococcus,* and *P aeruginosa*, but cultures are often negative as a result of the patient's previous antibiotic therapy.

Common clinical symptoms include persistent fever, headache, and purulent otorrhea. Associated symptoms include ataxia, vomiting, and an altered level of consciousness that may present as drowsiness, lethargy, or mild disorientation [23]. If meningitis is present, symptoms may also include photophobia and nuchal rigidity. Many of the symptoms associated with suppurative intracranial complications have been discussed previously with complications related to sinusitis.

Another rare complication of otitis media is Gradenigo's syndrome, which describes a constellation of symptoms that occur secondary to inflammation of the petrous apex. The petrous apex surrounds the internal auditory canal and can become infected easily because the air cells that compose its structure communicate with the middle ear cleft. It occurs most commonly as a complication of chronic otitis media, with long-standing purulent otorrhea. Gradenigo's syndrome exists when infection of the petrous apex is associated with a sixth nerve palsy, otorrhea, and retro-orbital pain [24]. Because infection may often spread unchecked, deficits in cranial nerves II through XII also may occur. Because of this presentation, the clinician should be alert to symptoms of Bell's palsy in the presence of an inner ear infection.

The initial procedure of choice to diagnose intracranial complications is CT with intravenous contrast. In addition to providing detailed images of the bony structures, CT also can indicate the presence of space-occupying lesions. If meningitis is suspected, a lumbar puncture should be performed once the risk of herniation can be eliminated.

Lateral sinus thrombosis

Lateral (transverse) sinus thrombosis results from septic thrombophlebitis or a direct infectious extension from the mastoid bone and is the third most common intracranial complications of otitis media [25]. Because of the patient's previous antibiotic therapy, the clinical presentation may be variable, but most patients will complain of a unilateral occipital or temporal headache that was preceded by an ear infection or otalgia by several weeks [22]. Other symptoms may include fever, nausea, vomiting, vertigo, and altered mental status [26]. The physical examination may reveal an abnormal ear examination, papilledema, mastoid tenderness, cranial nerve palsies, posterior auricular swelling, and nuchal rigidity [27].

Complicated pharyngeal infections: epiglottitis

Acute epiglottitis is a potentially life-threatening condition that results from inflammation of the supraglottic structures. Commonly thought of as a pediatric affliction, the current incidence of epiglottitis in adults is 0.97 to 1.8 per 100,000, which exceeds the incidence in children by 2.5 times [28]. Currently, the most common cause of epiglottitis is infection, but other sources such as crack cocaine use have also been implicated [29]. Common pathogens include *H influenzae*, β-hemolytic streptococci, and viruses.

The "classic" symptoms of epiglottitis are sore throat, odynophagia, acute onset of fever, stridor, and drooling. Unfortunately, these rarely occur simultaneously in the adult patient. One review has noted that "classic" symptoms were rarely present together and that the symptoms did not present acutely but rather over a period of several days [30]. Furthermore, an elevated temperature was also rarely present. The lack of symptoms often leads to a misdiagnosis. It is estimated that a diagnosis is made in 35% to 70% of cases during the initial physician evaluation [31,32]. The most common clinical findings in adults are sore throat, odynophagia, a muffled voice, and pharyngitis accompanied by anterior neck tenderness [33].

A high index of suspicion for epiglottitis should be present in any patient who presents with a chief complaint of a severe sore throat. The suspicion should be raised further if the patient experiences extreme discomfort on palpation of the larynx [34]. The physician should also entertain the possibility of other conditions, which may mimic epiglottitis, such as angioneurotic edema, foreign bodies, trauma, and infections such as diphtheria, pertussis, and croup.

Examination through direct laryngoscopic visualization of the epiglottis is the definitive diagnosis. If epiglottitis is suspected, the patient should be transferred by ambulance to an emergency department or facility with the capabilities to safely visualize the epiglottis and obtain a surgical airway if compromise develops. CT also may be performed if a laryngoscopic evaluation cannot be performed or if coexistent soft tissue complications are suspected.

Deep neck infections

The organs and vascular, neurologic, and structural elements of the neck are invested and bound together by fibrous cervical fascia. This subdivides the neck into functional components and creates tissue planes that extend the length and width of the neck (Fig. 1). In the nonpathologic state, these potential spaces are present as loose connective tissue that can become eroded easily by infection or tumor infiltration.

Structurally, the hyoid bone acts as a barrier to infection and serves as an anatomic landmark into which the deep compartments can be subdivided. The compartments can be separated into those existing above, below, and in the plane of the hyoid bone (anatomic landmarks are discussed with each clinical entity). Although a number of deep tissue compartments exist, the three most significant areas are the submandibular, retropharyngeal, and parapharyngeal spaces.

These spaces are clearly delineated anatomic compartments, but they communicate freely with each other and allow for the easy spread of infections and tumors. Deep tissue infections can result from a contiguous source as in the case of Ludwig's angina or from lymphatic spread in retropharyngeal space infection. Other sources of infection include trauma from intravenous drug use, sialadenitis, suppurative lymphadenitis, or the infection of a pre-existing cyst. What begins as a localized infection can turn into a deep tissue infection, causing complications such as mediastinitis, cavernous sinus thrombosis, internal jugular thrombophlebitis, and carotid artery dissection [35–37].

Although the majority of patients will present with classic findings such as neck swelling, trismus, and signs of septic instability, some patients, such as the elderly and immunocompromised, may present with more subtle symptoms [38]. The challenge is to identify the patient who has subtle symptoms of deep tissue infection to prevent the significant complications that may occur.

Peritonsillar abscess

Peritonsillar abscess (PTA) has been clinically documented since the 1700s, but a general description of the disease can be traced to Celsus in

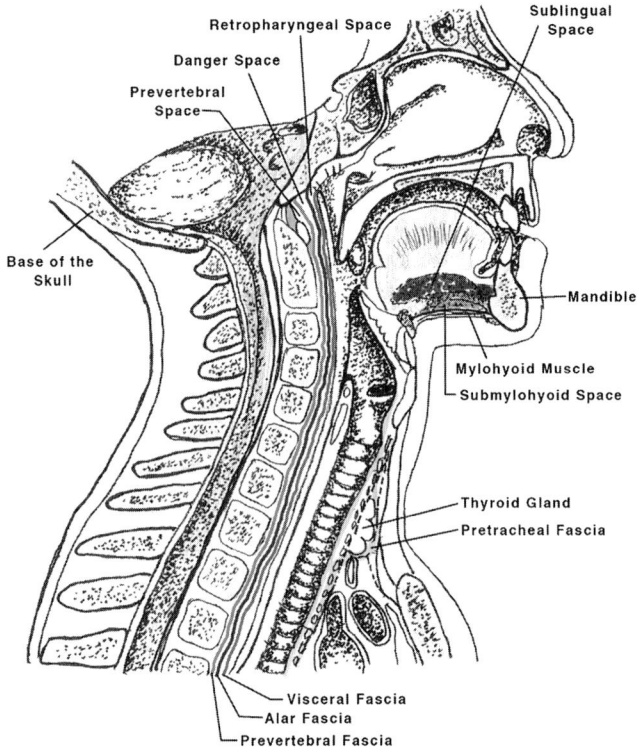

Fig. 1. Functional components of the neck. (Courtesy of Jocelyn Belleza.)

the second and third century BC. Despite the use of antibiotics for the treatment of tonsillitis and pharyngitis, PTA remains the most common abscess of the head and neck [39]. Left untreated, PTA can spread through the deep tissues and produce complications such as airway compromise, mediastinitis, thrombophlebitis, and hemorrhage from involvement of the submaxillary arteries [39–41].

PTA commonly affects young adults between the age of 15 and 30 and most commonly occurs from November to December and April to May, a time frame that coincides with the highest incidences of streptococcal pharyngitis and exudative tonsillitis.

PTA has been classically conceived of as the endpoint of a continuum that begins with an acute exudative tonsillitis that progresses to cellulitis and, eventually, to abscess formation. A recent review [42] points to the role of Weber's glands, which are salivary glands located in the supratonsillar fossa, in the formation of peritonsillar abscesses. It is believed that the supratonsillar space first becomes inflamed, which leads to the development of cellulitis. As the infection progresses, the tissue planes between the tonsil and its surrounding aponeurosis become obliterated, resulting in scarring and ductal obstruction of Weber's glands. Increasing ductal obstruction results eventually in glandular obstruction and, if untreated, results in abscess formation. It is this abscess formation and inflammation that produces the classical symptoms of PTA.

Patients who have PTA will present with complaints of fever, severe sore throat, discomfort at the angle of the jaw, odynophagia, and otalgia Physical findings may reveal a drooling patient with a partially opened mouth, speaking in a "hot potato" or muffled voice that results from transient dysfunction of the palatal muscles.

Examination usually reveals trismus, with the patient unable to open his or her mouth more than 2.5 cm. The oropharynx appears erythematous, with a darker area of unilateral redness overlying the involved side and a tense swelling of the anterior pillar and soft palate above the involved tonsil (Fig. 2). The uvula and the tonsil may be displaced by the abscess. PTA may be difficult to distinguish from other common processes such as peritonsillar cellulitis, retromolar abscesses, and infectious mononucleosis. The presence of a longer prodromal period and lack of fluctuance distinguish infectious mononucleosis from a PTA (Fig. 3), whereas the presence of significant dental caries may indicate the presence of a retromolar abscess. Peritonsillar cellulitis is extremely difficult to discriminate clinically from PTA and may be distinguished by the lack of purulent material during a needle aspiration.

If PTA is suspected, the patient should be referred immediately to the emergency department or an otolaryngologist for specialized care and possible airway management. The definitive therapy for PTA requires

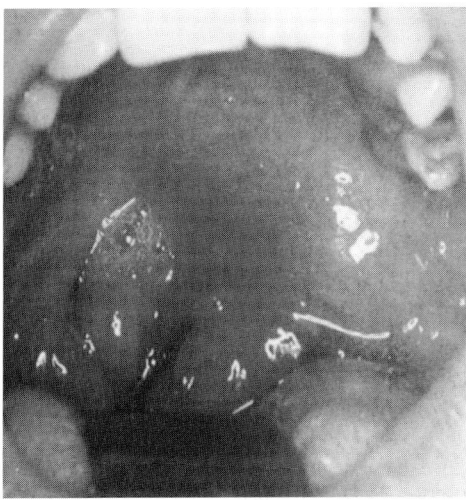

Fig. 2. Intraoral view of peritonsillar abscess. (Courtesy of Joydeep Som, MD.)

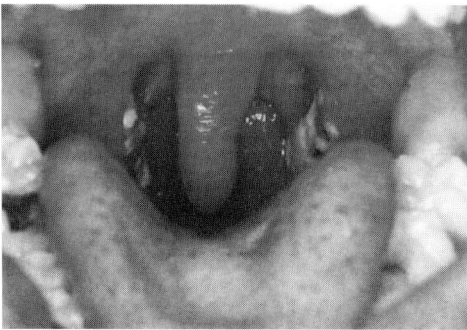

Fig. 3. Intraoral view of infectious mononucleosis. (Courtesy of Joydeep Som, MD.)

administration of broad-spectrum antibiotics and drainage of the abscess. Because the microbiology of these infections is polymicrobial and predominantly anaerobic [43], antibiotic choices include a combination of penicillin and β-lactamase inhibitor or carbapenem, chloramphenicol, or clindamycin.

Although some studies point to the efficacy of outpatient treatment with needle aspiration [44], other studies report a higher rate of abscess recurrence compared with incision and drainage [45]. In addition, needle aspiration has been associated with a false-negative rate of up to 24% [46,47] and can be complicated by laceration of the carotid artery [48]. A recent evidence-based review of treatment options indicates that both modalities have had equal success and the evidence supports the use of either treatment [49]. Because of the difficulty in definitively diagnosing PTA clinically, the potential for airway compromise, the possible adverse effects of unguided needle aspiration, and the lack of adequate oral antimicrobial agents, the present authors recommend the patient be admitted to an inpatient setting or an emergency department with the capability obtaining a surgical airway.

Ludwig's angina

Ludwig's angina was first documented by Wilhelm Frederick von Ludwig in 1836 as a gangrenous induration involving the connective tissue of the neck and floor of the mouth. The tissue space involved is the submandibular space, which is subdivided into the sublingual and submylohyoid spaces. Both spaces are bounded superiorly by the floor of the mouth, base of the tongue, and the ramus of the mandible. The floor of this space is created by the mylohyoid muscle, the hyoid bone, and the posterior belly of the digastric muscle. Both spaces communicate with each other as well as with the pharyngomaxillary and retropharyngeal spaces. Infectious expansion into the space occurs superiorly and posteriorly because of the mandible and mylohyoid muscle, which limit anterior and inferior extension. As a result, unchecked infections that extend into the floor of the mouth can compromise the oral cavity and airway and spread toward the deep neck spaces and the mediastinum.

An odontogenic focus is the source of infection in 85% of Ludwig's angina cases, with patients reporting either a history of recent dental work or dental pain [50]. The second and third molars are the most common odontogenic foci. Other sources include peritonsillar abscesses, oral malignancy, and mandibular fractures [51–53]. Predisposing factors include dental caries, sickle cell diseases, immunocompromised states, and trauma [54]. The most common causative agents are *Streptococcus*, *Staphylococcus*, and *Bacteroides* species.

Ludwig's angina usually begins as a mild infection that rapidly progresses, in which most patients present with brawny neck swelling, tongue protrusion, and severe pain [50,55]. Other complaints include trismus, fever, malaise, and a fetid breath. Trismus is present if the masticator muscles are involved but may not be present if the infection has spread posteriorly.

Although one fourth of patients will present with signs of respiratory compromise, the physician should examine for signs of swelling in the floor of the mouth in any patient complaining of neck pain. If a patient is suspected of having Ludwig's angina, supplemental oxygen should be given, and the patient should be transported by ambulance to a facility with the capacity to obtain a possible surgical airway. Definitive treatment requires the administration of broad-spectrum antibiotics, debridement, and drainage in the operating room.

Parapharyngeal space infection

The parapharyngeal space is also known as the pharyngomaxillary or lateral pharyngeal space. Structurally, it can be thought of as an inverted cone, with its base formed by the petrous bone and the apex at the hyoid bone. It can be further subdivided into an anterior and posterior compartment, with specific signs and symptoms for the compartment involved.

Sources of infection include the teeth, pharynx, tonsils, the middle ear, parotid glands, and lymph glands. The most common presenting symptoms are neck swelling and neck pain [56]. Anterior compartment involvement is characterized by irritation of the internal pterygoid muscle, producing trismus. If swelling occurs in the area of the epiglottis or larynx, dyspnea may be present. Posterior compartment involvement produces minimal trismus but produces signs of sepsis or neurologic deficits (unilateral tongue paresis, hoarseness, and Horner syndrome) because of the proximity to the carotid sheath [57,58]. Another potential vascular complication is suppurative jugular thrombophlebitis. Symptoms include systemic toxicity and neck pain that occurs when turning the head *toward* the uninvolved side. This is caused by compression of the infected area by the sternocleidomastoid muscle.

Physical findings include systemic toxicity and medial deviation of the lateral pharyngeal wall and tonsil. One study [59] has demonstrated that the most common finding in patients with parapharyngeal abscess was nonfluctuant swelling at the angle of the mandible. Unfortunately, these symptoms may not be present in the older or immunocompromised adult. One study [38] of older adults has demonstrated that fever and toxicity were rarely present, and the most common findings were pharyngeal asymmetry and pharyngitis. Definitive treatment requires hospital admission, aggressive antibiotic therapy, and incision and drainage in the operating room.

Retropharyngeal space infection

The retropharyngeal space is a potential space bordered posteriorly by the prevertebral fascia and anteriorly by the pharyngeal muscle and its fascia. Its superior border is the base of the skull, and its inferior border is formed by the fascial fusion of the previously mentioned anterior and posterior components. The retropharyngeal space is considered a "danger" space because of its close proximity to the vertebral structures and direct communication with the mediastinum.

Retropharyngeal abscess (RPA) occurs more commonly in children and, until recently, has been an uncommon entity in the adult [60]. Some reports [55] have noted an increasing incidence of this entity in adults.

In children, the formation of an RPA is believed to be secondary to suppuration of retropharyngeal nodes that are seeded from a distant infection. These nodes regress in the adult, which may explain the relative infrequency among older patients. In adults, RPA usually is caused by infectious spread from the previously mentioned deep spaces or from local invasion. Local invasion occurs typically from the violation of the mucosa by cervical spine trauma, foreign bodies, and procedural instrumentation [61]. As a result, one of the early symptoms of RPA is a progressively worsening sore throat after instrumentation of the oropharynx or gastrointestinal tract.

RPA can be diagnosed by a lateral soft tissue radiograph of the neck. A retropharyngeal diameter greater than 7 mm at C2 or 22 mm at C6 is considered abnormal and supports the diagnosis of an RPA [62]. As with other deep tissue abscesses, definitive treatment requires surgical drainage and directed antibiotic therapy.

Foreign bodies

Foreign bodies in the nose and ear

Although they are not life threatening, foreign bodies retained in the nose and ear may produce discomfort and agitation and result in secondary complications such infection and mucosal erosion. Unlike foreign bodies in children, foreign bodies in adults are inserted deliberately in an effort to clean, relieve irritation, and control bleeding in the ear and nose. In adults, the majority of foreign bodies are inanimate (paper, cotton swabs, or sponge material), but live objects such as insects, larvae, and worms may be encountered occasionally.

The most common location for foreign bodies in the nasal cavity is below the inferior turbinate or anterior to the middle turbinate. If the patient is cooperative, direct visualization is easily accomplished and essential for proper removal of a foreign body. Visualization requires a good light source, preferably from a headlamp, and a nasal speculum.

The majority of items are retrievable using grasping instruments such as straight forceps, alligator forceps, and mosquito clamps. If an object is small, alligator forceps may be inserted through an otoscope head to aid in visualization. Other methods include suction, irrigation, and adhesives. Irrigation and wash techniques should be avoided if the object is vegetative or prone to further expansion if wet or if the patient is at risk for aspiration. If a living object is encountered, it must be killed or stunned before removal. The patient should be examined by an otolaryngologist or emergency physician if he or she cannot cooperate, if removal may produce further obstruction or aspiration, and if infection or extensive tissue destruction is present.

If a patient presents with a retained foreign body in the external auditory canal, the physician should first evaluate for signs for secondary complications such as hearing loss, nystagmus, vertigo, cranial nerve deficits, or deep-seated infection. If these are present, immediate consultation with an otolaryngologist is required. Unlike foreign bodies in the nose, direct visualization of the external ear canal may be difficult because of the anatomic nature of the canal and secondary inflammatory or traumatic changes. The patient should also be referred to an otolaryngologist or emergency room if the foreign body cannot be visualized, is deeply impacted, or the patient is unable to cooperate.

The primary means of removing a foreign body in the ear are irrigation, suction, and direct visualization. Irrigation is accomplished using an 18-gauge catheter attached to a 10- to 20-mL syringe. The flow of fluid should be directed around the retained object, which will allow backpressure to force the object out of the canal. Fluids should be close to body temperature to avoid irritation of the labyrinths. Irrigation should be avoided if it will result in further expansion of the object. Continuous suction may be used, especially if the object has a smooth contour. Direct instrumentation can be attempted in the same fashion as with nasal foreign bodies. Once again, instrumentation should be performed only if the object can be visualized directly. Complications include laceration of the external canal and, rarely, perforation of the tympanic membrane.

Foreign bodies in the esophagus

Foreign bodies may become entrapped in the esophagus by accidental (dentures or teeth) or intentional ingestion (food impaction). Although patients with high-grade obstructions and compromise are more likely to present to an emergency department, primary care physicians may still encounter patients with symptoms of partial obstruction or foreign body sensation.

The history should concentrate on the likely agent and the duration of symptoms. The initial physical examination should focus on signs of compromise or secondary complications. Although drooling and stridor indicate impending compromise, findings such as crepitation, neck tenderness, and fever may be signs of esophageal perforation. Patients demonstrating these symptoms or who report entrapment for 24 hours or greater should be transferred to an emergency department by ambulance.

The esophagus has three areas of physiologic narrowing, located at the upper esophageal sphincter, the aortic arch, and the diaphragmatic hiatus, which may provide foci for entrapment. In patients who have esophageal pathology, foreign bodies may became entrapped at these areas or other points of pathologic stricture. Once stability has been assured, the history should seek to locate the likely location of obstruction by symptoms. The secondary physical examination should begin with an examination of the pharynx and hypopharynx for signs of the foreign body, a clue to its origin (missing tooth or denture plate), and abrasions that may mimic symptoms of a foreign body.

Unfortunately, the physical examination is often unrevealing, so further radiologic imaging by plain radiography or CT scanning is required. Management strategies vary and require the aid of a gastroenterologist in a monitored setting. Methods depend on the nature of the foreign body (meat impaction or animal bone, sharp or dull), the level of entrapment, and the risk that it may produce perforation or erosion. The only patients who would be eligible for discharge from the office with expectant treatment are those who are not experiencing evidence of obstruction or secondary complications (perforation) and those who have ingested "low risk" objects (eg, coins) that have already passed into the stomach. Before discharge, passage into the stomach should be confirmed radiographically, and follow-up care should be arranged with the primary physician or a gastroenterologist.

Orbit trauma

Patients suffering significant facial trauma generally present to emergency departments and trauma centers. However, the primary care physician may encounter patients who have less severe injuries, often with delayed presentations. Obtaining a relevant history and performing a focused physical examination are essential for recognizing conditions that will necessitate referral to an emergency department or specialist. Additionally, interventions easily performed in the office setting serve as a definitive treatment or a temporizing measure until the patient can be transferred to an emergency department.

Although this section focuses on the ENT aspects of trauma, the primary care physician should recognize that over 50% of facial trauma is associated with other injuries [6]. Hopefully and likely, patients with cardiac instability or airway compromise will be transported directly to an emergency department. However, patients with less obvious but potentially dangerous injuries may present to a primary care office. The examination should begin with a full set of vital signs, followed by a history regarding the mechanism and time of trauma, which may point toward likely injury patterns. Inquiring about the mechanism of injury is particularly important in female patients and children, who are more frequently victims of domestic violence and abuse. The physician should also inquire about loss of consciousness following the injury because this may signify intracranial pathology.

The physical examination should include cardiac and pulmonary auscultation, abdominal palpation, and neurovascular examination. The patient's cervical spine should be evaluated. Patients with midline tenderness and a significant mechanism for injury should be placed in rigid collar and referred to the emergency department for further evaluation. After confirming that the patient is stable, a more focused examination of the head can proceed.

A simple visual assessment of the face can reveal areas of concern. The physician should evaluate the face for asymmetry and deformity. Sensory examination should include testing of the three distributions of the trigeminal nerve. Motor function of both the upper and lower face (cranial nerve VII) can be assessed by having the patient wrinkle the forehead, smile, bare the teeth, and close the eyes tightly [63]. Although a thorough ophthalmologic examination is beyond the scope of this article, visual acuity should be documented.

Orbital wall fractures typically result from mechanisms of low to moderate force, commonly the result of a direct blow during an altercation [64]. The medial wall and the orbital floor are the most susceptible to fracture. Significant disruption of these bony structures can result in entrapment of the medial or inferior rectus muscles.

The orbits should be carefully inspected for deformity or asymmetry. Proptosis and enophthalmos suggest a complete orbital rim blowout fracture and are associated with significant mechanisms of trauma. Areas of concern should be gently palpated for tenderness, step-offs, and crepitus. Evaluation of motor and sensory function should follow. Sensory deficits in the distribution of the infraorbital nerve (cranial nerve V) are associated with the disruption of the inferior orbital wall. Extra ocular muscles should be evaluated; pain or diplopia with movement, as well as inability to move the eye, may signify muscle entrapment. Any concern for an orbital wall fracture should prompt referral or transport to an emergency department for appropriate imaging and possible consultation with both ophthalmology and otolaryngology specialists.

Ear

The examination should begin with questioning the patient about subjective hearing loss or tinnitus. Performing Weber's and Rinne's tests can provide responses that distinguish between conductive and sensorineural hearing loss [65]. The physician should then carefully examine the external ear for evidence of hematoma (Fig. 4). An untreated auricular hematoma can lead to development of "cauliflower ear". After draining the hematoma with needle aspiration or a small linear incision, the physician should apply a pressure bandage to prevent the reaccumulation of blood. The evaluation of the external auditory meatus and tympanic membrane should follow an external examination of the ear. Patients who have a disrupted tympanic membrane or an impaled foreign object should be referred to an otolaryngologist for further evaluation.

Nose

Motor vehicle collisions and assaults account for the majority of nasal traumas. Nondisplaced nasal fractures generally do not require immediate intervention and can be referred for ENT follow-up in 3 to 5 days. However, for fractures caused by proximity, coexistent intracranial trauma must be excluded. Cerebrospinal fluid (CSF) rhinorrhea signifies damage to the cribriform plate and requires urgent neurosurgical evaluation. Testing the glucose level in the fluid may distinguish simple nasal secretions (low

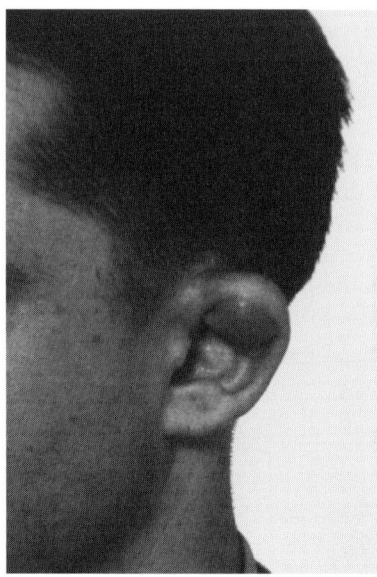

Fig. 4. Presentation of auricular hematoma. (Courtesy of Joydeep Som, MD.)

glucose) from CSF (high glucose). The presence of a double ring when bloody nasal fluid is placed on filter paper may also indicate the presence of CSF. However, the current literature does not support the use of glucose testing or filter paper, secondary to poor sensitivity and specificity. The β_2 transferrin assay is the test of choice for confirming CSF leakage [66]. Any concern for CSF leakage (including otorrhea) should prompt transport to the emergency department for a definitive diagnosis.

Epistaxis is associated frequently with nasal trauma. Bleeding can occur from anterior and posterior sources. Bleeding from Kiesselbach's plexus (anterior) occurs most commonly; direct, continuous pressure for 10 to 15 minutes generally halts further bleeding. If direct pressure proves unsuccessful, silver nitrate sticks serve to cauterize the source of anterior bleeding. Commercially marketed nasal tampons (eg, Merocel; Medtronic, Mystic, Connecticut) also halt anterior bleeds through a compression mechanism and are generally left in the nares for 3 to 5 days. Patients with nasal packing should receive prophylactic antibiotics to avoid toxic shock [63,67].

Patients who have posterior epistaxis can lose large volumes of blood and are at risk for cardiovascular compromise, without intervention. Posterior nosebleeds originate from the sphenopalatine artery and always require otolaryngology consultation for definitive treatment. As a temporizing measure, the physician can pass a Foley catheter through the nostril into the oral cavity, inflate the balloon, and then gently pull backward on the catheter. Passing a balloon is contraindicated in patients who have significant facial trauma or clear evidence of CSF rhinorrhea. All patients who have posterior nosebleeds require immediate transfer to an emergency department. Symptomatic patients or those at increased risk for hemodynamic compromise (ie, history of angina) require the placement of a large-bore intravenous line and monitored transport.

The physician should also evaluate the nares for a septal hematoma. The easily identifiable hematoma (resembling a bulging grape) should be drained with a small horizontal incision. Drainage prevents avascular necrosis of the septum and corresponding "saddle nose" deformity. As with patients who have anterior epistaxis, the physician should pack the nares and prescribe antibiotics.

Mandible

When assessing the mandible, the physician should inquire whether the patient has been able to open and close his or her mouth normally. Instructing the patient to bite firmly on a tongue depressor on both sides of the mouth effectively tests temporomandibular joint integrity. The oral cavity should be inspected for evidence of trauma or missing teeth. Gentle pressure should be applied to teeth to assess laxity. Patients who have malocclusion, dental laxity, or trauma should be referred to an emergency department for consultation with a maxillofacial specialist.

Patient who have facial trauma will occasionally present to their primary care physician in lieu of an emergency department. A brief but thorough history and physical examination can identify patients who will require further evaluation and treatment. Red flags, including midline cervical spine tenderness, signs of extra ocular muscle entrapment, CSF rhinorrhea, and malocclusion of the mandible should prompt expedited transport to an emergency department.

Ear, nose, and throat complications of body piercing

Image enhancement by body piercing has been a centuries old practice performed by various cultures throughout the world. More recently, in the latter half of the twentieth century, piercing of nontraditional areas of the body (tongue and genitalia) has become commonplace, especially among young adults. In addition to these nontraditional areas, the increasing use of the upper third of the pinna has resulted in a new variety of local cartilaginous and systemic complications not seen formerly by the clinician.

Perichondritis

Cartilage is avascular and requires metabolic support from the adherent perichondrium. Transcartilaginous piercing, performed most commonly with multiuse ear piercing guns, results in traumatic disruption of the cartilaginous–perichondrial relationship. In addition, piercing allows for the introduction of local microflora into an otherwise sterile and poorly vascularized subcutaneous area.

Perichondritis results from an infection of the cartilage and subcutaneous tissue by pathogens such as *P aeruginosa* and *Staph aureus*. *Pseudomonas* organisms have been implicated in the majority of documented perichondritis cases [68]. Other organisms identified include *Streptococcus*, *Proteus*, and *Lactobacillus* species. This infection is more commonplace in the summer months when excessive perspiration may inhibit proper healing [69]. Early clinical features of perichondritis include pain, erythema, and local warmth that usually occur 3 to 4 weeks after implantation and will often develop before swelling begins. The formation of a subperiosteal abscess results in the destructive loss of cartilage and the structural support for the pinna (Fig. 5). This structural disruption can result in the formation of the deformity commonly known as cauliflower ear, which is often recalcitrant to reconstruction.

Because transcartilaginous infections spread rapidly and can lead to severe cosmetic deformity, early and aggressive therapy is required. Antibiotics should be instituted when infection is first suspected and should be broad enough to eradicate both *Pseudomonas* spp and *Staph aureus*. Fluoroquinolones and intravenous antipseudomonal penicillins are appropriate agents.

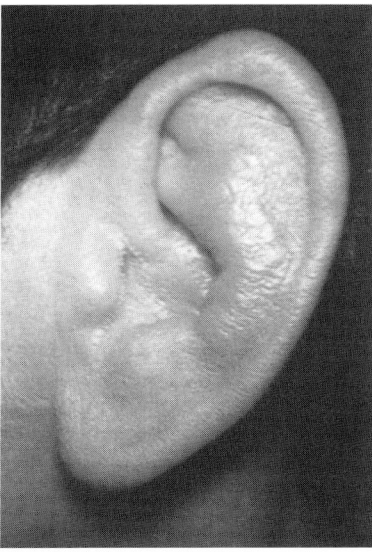

Fig. 5. Presentation of auricular perichondritis. (Courtesy of Joydeep Som, MD.)

Admission and early surgical intervention are required at signs of systemic toxicity, abscess formation, or if the patient is immunocompromised.

Physicians should maintain a high level of vigilance for outbreaks of auricular perichondritis. An outbreak of pseudomonal-induced perichondritis occurred in Oregon, in 2000, as the result of pathogenic colonization of the disinfectant and the facilities at a jewelry kiosk [70]. The increasing popularity of upper ear piercing, lack of regulatory control, and the performance of the procedure by unlicensed and poorly trained personnel could lead to further outbreaks in the future.

Tongue piercing

As with the case of transcartilaginous piercing, piercing of the tongue, nose, and lip has been increasing in popularity. Fortunately, complications related to these procedures are relatively minor and include hypersensitivity reactions, granulomatous formation, local gingival and dental trauma, and difficulties with phonation, swallowing, and sensation.

Transmissible infections such as hepatitis and herpes simplex can be avoided if proper sterile technique is used by adequately trained personnel. More severe infections from invasion by microflora can result if a localized infection spreads along fascial planes. One reported complication of tongue piercing is a case of Ludwig's angina [71]. The presence of edema, erythema, and crepitation should prompt an expeditious referral to an emergency department.

Summary

Disease processes involving the ear, nose, and throat account for millions of office visits to primary care physicians per year. Because of their proximity to the airway as well as critical neurologic and vascular structures, the disease process in each individual case carries the potential for significant complications. Fortunately, improvements in medical care have significantly reduced the prevalence of these complications.

As a result of their relative rarity, most physicians may be unfamiliar with the clinical presentation of these entities. This article familiarizes the physician with the pathophysiology and clinical presentation of the more commonly encountered otolaryngologic complications. The physician should seek to rule out the presence of the aforementioned complications in each patient who presents with an otolaryngologic complaint. Any suggestion of their presence should prompt an immediate referral to a subspecialist or an emergency department. It is hoped that continued familiarization with these disease processes will maintain them as rare entities of medical practice.

References

[1] Wispelwey B, Dacey RG Jr, Scheld WM. Brain abscesses. In: Scheld WM, Whitley RJ, Durack DT, editors. Infections of the central nervous system. New York: Raven Press; 1991.
[2] UpToDate. Putting clinical information into practice. Galtne JM. Acute sinusitis and rhinosinusitis. Available at: http://www.uptodate.com. Accessed December 2004.
[3] Smith AT, Spencer JF. Orbital complications resulting from lesions of sinuses. Ann Otol Rhinol Laryngol 1948;57:5–27.
[4] Chandler JR, Langenbrunner DJ, Stevens ER. The pathogenesis of orbital complications in acute sinusitis. Laryngoscope 1970;80:1414–28.
[5] Howe L, Jones NS. Guidelines for the management of periorbital cellulitis/abscess. Clin Otolaryngol 2004;29:725–8.
[6] Ferguson MP, McNab AA. Current treatment and outcome in orbital cellulitis. Aust N Z J Ophthalmol 1999;27:375–9.
[7] Jackson K, Baker SR. Periorbital cellulitis. Head Neck Surg 1987;9:227–34.
[8] Marshall AH, Jones NS. Osteomyelitis of the frontal bone secondary to frontal sinusitis. J Laryngol Otol 2000;114:944–6.
[9] DiNubile MJ. Septic thrombosis of the cavernous sinuses. Arch Neurol 1988;45:567.
[10] Ebright JR, Pace MT, Niazi AF. Septic thrombosis of the cavernous sinuses. Arch Intern Med 2001;161(22):2671–6.
[11] Schuknecht B, Simmen D, Yuskel C, et al. Tributary venosinus occlusion and septic cavernous sinus thrombosis: CT and MRI findings. AJNR Am J Neuroradiol 1998;19:617–26.
[12] Dolan RW, Chowdury K. Diagnosis and treatment of intracranial complications of paranasal sinus infections. J Oral Maxillofac Surg 1995;53:1080–7.
[13] Jones NS, Walker JL, Bassi S, et al. The intracranial complications of rhinosinusitis: can they be prevented? Laryngoscope 2002;112(1):59–63.
[14] Gallagher RM, Gross CW, Phillips CD. Suppurative intracranial complications of sinusitis. Laryngoscope 1998;108:1635–42.

[15] Wispelway B. Brain abscesses. In: Mandell GL, Bleck TB, editors. Atlas of infectious diseases: central nervous system and eye infections. volume 13. New York: Churchill Livingstone; 1995. p. 887–900.
[16] Cassisi N, Cohn A, Davidson T, et al. Diffuse otitis externa; clinical and microbiological findings in the course of a multicenter study on a new otic solution. Ann Otol Rhinol Laryngol 1977;96(3 Pt 3)(Suppl 39):S1–16.
[17] UpToDate. Putting clinical information into practice. Klein JO. Epidemiology, pathogenesis, diagnosis, and complications of otitis media. Available at: http://www.uptodate.com. Accessed December 2004.
[18] Rubin J, Yu VL. Malignant external otitis: insights into pathogenesis, clinical manifestations, diagnosis, and therapy. Am J Med 1988;85:391–8.
[19] Handzel O, Halperin D. Necrotizing (malignant) external otitis. Am Fam Physician 2003; 68(2):309–12.
[20] Osma U, Cureoglu S, Hosoglu S. The complications of chronic otitis media: report of 93 cases. J Laryngol Otol 2000;114:97–100.
[21] Penido Nde O, Borin A, Iha LC, et al. Intracranial complications of otitis media: 15 years of experience in 33 patients. Otolaryngol Head Neck Surg 2005;132(1):37–42.
[22] Heilpern KL, Lorber B. Focal intracranial infections. Inf Dis Clin North Am 1996;10(4): 879–98.
[23] Sennaroglu L, Sozeri B. Otogenic brain abscesses: review of 41 cases. Otolaryngol Head Neck Surg 2000;123(6):751–5.
[24] Sherman SC, Buchanan A. Gradenigo syndrome: a case report and review of a rare complication of otitis media. J Emerg Med 2004;27(3):253–6.
[25] Kangsanarak J, Navacharoen N, Fooanant S, et al. Intracranial complications of suppurative otitis media: 13 years experience. Am J Otol 1995;16:104–9.
[26] Seven H, Ozbal AE, Turgut S. Management of otogenic lateral sinus thrombosis. Am J Otolaryngol 2004;25(5):329–33.
[27] Syms MJ, Tsai P, Holtel MR. Management of lateral sinus thrombosis. Laryngoscope 1999; 109(10):1616–20.
[28] Berg S, Trollfors B, Nylen O, et al. Incidence, aetiology, and prognosis of acute epiglottitis in children and adults in Sweden. Scand J Infect Dis 1996;28(3):261–4.
[29] Savitt DL, Colagiovanni S. Crack cocaine-related epiglottitis. Ann Emerg Med 1991;20: 322–3.
[30] Singer JI, McCabe J. Epiglottitis at the extremes of age. Am J Emerg Med 1988;6(3):228–31.
[31] Sheikh KH, Mostow SR. Epiglottitis—an increasing problem for adults. West J Med 1989; 151:520–4.
[32] Fontanarosa PB, Polsky SS, Goldman GE. Adult epiglottitis. J Emerg Med 1989;7:223–31.
[33] Sack JL, Brock CD. Identifying acute epiglottitis in adults. Postgrad Med 2002;112(1):81–2.
[34] Carey M. Epiglottitis in adults. Am J Emerg Med 1996;14(4):421–4.
[35] Harbour RC, Jonathan JD, Ballinger WE. Septic cavernous sinus thrombosis associated with gingivitis and parapharyngeal abscess. Arch Ophthalmol 1984;102:94–7.
[36] Eliachar I, Peleg H, Jochims HZ. Mediastinitis and bilateral pyopneumothorax complicating a parapharyngeal abscess. Head Neck Surg 1981;3:438–42.
[37] el-Sayed Y, al Dousary SA. Deep-neck space abscesses. J Otolaryngol 1996;25(4):227–33.
[38] Franzese CB, Isaacson JE. Peritonsillar and parapharyngeal space abscess in the older adult. Am J Otolaryngol 2003;24:169–73.
[39] Civen R, Vaisanen ML, Finegold SM. Peritonsillar abscess, retropharyngeal abscess, mediastinitis, and nonclostridial myonecrosis: a case report. Clin Infect Dis 1993;16(Suppl 4): S299–303.
[40] Epperly TD, Wood TC. New trends in the management of peritonsillar abscess. Am Fam Physician 1990;42(1):102–12.
[41] Wills PI, Vernon RP. Complications of space infections of the head and neck. Laryngoscope 1981;91:1129–36.

[42] Passy V. Pathogenesis of peritonsillar abscess. Laryngoscope 1994;104(2):185–90.
[43] Brook I. Microbiology and management of peritonsillar, retropharyngeal, and parapharyngeal abscesses. J Oral Maxillofac Surg 2004;62:1545–50.
[44] Ophir D, Bawnik J, Poria Y, et al. Peritonsillar abscess: a prospective evaluation of outpatient management by needle aspiration. Arch Otolaryngol Head Neck Surg 1988;114:661.
[45] Wolf M, Even-Chen I, Kronenberg J. Peritonsillar abscess: repeated needle aspiration versus incision and drainage. Ann Otol Rhinol Laryngol 1994;103:554–8.
[46] Spires JR, Ownes JJ, Woodson GE, et al. Treatment of peritonsillar abscess: a prospective study of aspiration vs. incision and drainage. Arch Otolaryngol Head Neck Surg 1987; 113:984–8.
[47] Buckley A, Moss E, Blokmanis A. Diagnosis of peritonsillar abscess: value of intraoral sonography. AJR Am J Roentgenol 1994;162:961–4.
[48] Lyon M, Glisson P, Blaivas M. Bilateral peritonsillar abscess diagnosed on the bases of intraoral sonography. J Ultrasound Med 2003;22:993–6.
[49] Johnson RF, Stewart MG, Wright CC. An evidence based review of the treatment of peritonsillar abscess. Otolaryngol Head Neck Surg 2003;128(3):332–43.
[50] Moreland LW, Corey J, McKenzie R. Ludwig's angina. Report of a case and review of the literature. Arch Intern Med 1988;148(2):461–6.
[51] Weisengreen HH. Ludwig's angina: historical review and reflections. Ear Nose Throat J 1986;65(10):457–61.
[52] Dreyer AF, de Kock SE, Rantloane JL. Ludwig's angina: a case report and review. J Dent Assoc S Afr 1990;45(9):397–400.
[53] Fischman GE, Graham BS. Ludwig's angina resulting from infection of an oral malignancy. J Oral Maxillofac Surg 1985;43:795–6.
[54] Hartman RW. Ludwig's angina in children. Am Fam Physician 1990;60(1):109–12.
[55] Sethi DS, Stanley RE. Deep neck abscesses-changing trends. J Laryngol Otol 1994;108: 138–43.
[56] Wang LF, Kuo WR, Tsai SM, et al. Characterizations of life-threatening deep cervical space infections: a review of one hundred ninety-six cases. Am J Otolaryngol 2003;24(2):111–7.
[57] Levitt GW. Cervical fascia and deep neck infections. Otolaryngol Clin North Am 1976;9(3): 703–16.
[58] UpToDate. Putting clinical information into practice. Chow AW. Peripharyngeal fascial space infections. Available at: http://www.uptodate.com. April 2003.
[59] Sethi DS, Stanley RE. Parapharyngeal abscesses. J Laryngol Otol 1991;105:1025–30.
[60] Tannenbaum RD. Adult retropharyngeal abscess: a case report and review of the literature. J Emerg Med 1996;14(2):147–58.
[61] Yen-Shuo T, Chung-Chung T. Retropharyngeal and epidural abscess from a swallowed fish bone. Am J Emerg Med 1997;15:381–3.
[62] Melio FR, Holmes DK. Upper respiratory infections. In: Rosen P, Barkin R, editors. Rosen's emergency medicine, concepts and clinical practice. 4th edition. St. Louis (MO): Mosby; 1998. p. 1529–42.
[63] Cantrell S. Face. In: Rosen's emergency medicine, concepts and clinical practice. 5th edition. St. Louis (MO): Mosby; 2002. p. 315–6.
[64] Seyfer AE, Hansen JE. Facial trauma. In: Mattox K, Feliciano D, Moore E, editors. Trauma. 4th edition. New York: McGraw-HIll; 1999. p. 415–33.
[65] Riviello R. Otolaryngologic procedures. In: Roberts J, Hedges J, editors. Clinical procedures in emergency medicine. Philadelphia: Elsevier; 2004. p. 1280–316.
[66] Chan DT, Poon WS, IP CP, et al. How useful is glucose detection in diagnosing cerebrospinal fluid leak? The rational use of CT and Beta-2 transferrin assay in detection of cerebrospinal fluid fistula. Asian J Surg 2004;27(1):39–42.
[67] Bandhauer F, Buhl D, Grossenbacher R. Antibiotic prophylaxis in rhinosurgery. Am J Rhinol 2002;16(3):135–9.
[68] George J, White M. Infection as a consequence of ear piercing. Practitioner 1989;23:404–6.

[69] Staley R, Fitzgibbon JJ, Anderson C. Auricular infections caused by high ear piercing in adolescents. Pediatrics 1997;99:610–1.
[70] Keene WE, Markum AC, Samadpour M. Outbreak of *Pseudomonas aeruginosa* infections caused by commercial piercing of upper ear cartilage. JAMA 2004;291(8):981–5.
[71] Perkins CS, Meisner J, Harrison J. A complication of tongue piercing. Br Dent J 1997;182: 147–8.

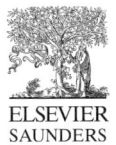

Orthopedic Trauma: Office Management of Major Joint Injury

Laura Pimentel, MD[a,b,*]

[a]Division of Emergency Medicine, University of Maryland School of Medicine, Baltimore, MD, USA
[b]Department of Emergency Medicine, Mercy Medical Center, Baltimore, MD, USA

Patients presenting with musculoskeletal pain and injury challenge the office internist with extensive differential diagnoses and management considerations. The acutely traumatized patient should be rapidly evaluated for the presence of life- or limb-threatening injuries. Any evidence of significant head, spinal, chest, abdominal, or pelvic injuries should precipitate rapid transfer to the closest emergency department. Similarly, patients who have open musculoskeletal trauma, obvious extremity deformity, or severe pain and those who are nonambulatory are better served in the emergency department than in the office.

Ambulatory patients who have isolated extremity pain or injury are appropriate candidates for office evaluation and treatment. Amadio and colleagues [1] compared care by primary care physicians with care by specialists and noted no difference in short-term outcome or patient satisfaction in patients who had knee injuries. A complete history and physical examination narrows the differential diagnosis and provides a working impression. Selected patients require imaging studies to confirm the correct diagnosis. The focus of this article is the clinical evaluation, diagnosis, and management of acute and subacute extremity injuries presenting to the outpatient setting.

The equipment and the supplies for management of orthopedic injuries vary from office to office depending on the patient population, location, proximity to a hospital emergency department, and availability of specialty consultation. Supplies to consider stocking in the office include elastic bandages, knee immobilizers, air casts, ankle stirrups, plaster or fiberglass splint material, canes, walkers, and crutches for lower-extremity injuries. Slings

---

* Department of Emergency Medicine, Mercy Medical Center, 301 St. Paul Place, Baltimore, MD 21228.
  E-mail address: lpiment@comcast.net

and preformed wrist splints should be considered for upper-extremity injuries. See Box 1 for general management principles for extremity fractures in the office.

Knee injuries

Acute traumatic injuries

The mechanism of injury is the most important aspect of the history in a patient who has acute knee trauma (Fig. 1). The mechanism should be categorized as the result of twisting, hyperextension, or a direct blow. Each has a discreet differential diagnosis. The presence of swelling and the acuity of onset should be ascertained. Other relevant historical features include location of the pain, hearing a "pop" at the time of injury, locking, and instability. Patients who have the primary complaint of knee pain may have referred pain from the low back or hip. History and examination directed to this possibility must be considered. General medical and surgical history should include rheumatologic diseases, medications, previous knee injuries, and knee surgery [2].

Physical examination is best conducted with the patient supine on the examining table. Long pants, shoes, and socks should be removed. Inspection

---

Box 1. Stable extremity fractures

1. Assess neurovascular status
2. Check for evidence of compartment syndrome (7 P's)
   - Pain out of proportion to injury[a]
   - Pain with passive extension of digits[a]
   - Pallor
   - Pulselessness
   - Paralysis
   - Paresthesias
   - Poikilothermia (cold extremity)
3. Ice
4. Elevation
5. Analgesics
6. Orthopedic follow-up care
7. Fractures
   - Upper-extremity: immobilize with splint, sling as appropriate
   - Lower-extremity: immobilize with splint, knee immobilizer as appropriate
8. Make patients non–weight bearing by fitting with crutches; consider walkers for elderly patients.

---

[a] Earliest and most sensitive findings.

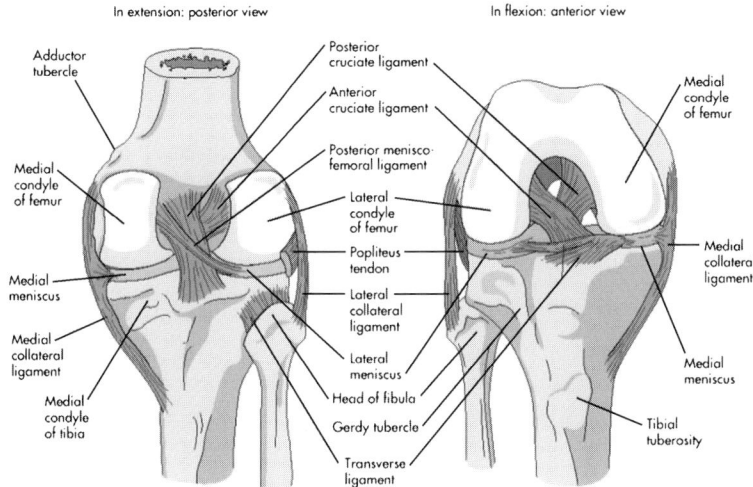

Fig. 1. Knee anatomy. (*From* Marx JA, Hockberger RS, Walls RM, editors. Rosen's emergency medicine: concepts and clinical practice. 5th edition. St. Louis (MO): Mosby; 2002. p. 675. Copyright © 2002 Mosby, Inc.; with permission.)

begins with comparison to the normal knee. The examiner looks for swelling, ecchymosis, erythema, and asymmetry. Range of motion should be assessed. The normal range extends from 0° in full extension to 135° when fully flexed. The patient should be asked to elevate the leg off the table to demonstrate integrity of the extensor mechanism. Palpation for point tenderness includes the patella, quadriceps tendon, patellar tendon, medial and lateral joint lines, tibial tubercle, and popliteal fossa [2]. Distal pulses should be checked. Stress testing of the knee primarily assesses ligamentous integrity and includes Lachman's test, anterior drawer, posterior drawer, and pivot shift maneuver. McMurray's test and the Apley compression test assess the meniscus [3].

Indications for plain radiographic imaging of patients who have acute knee trauma in the emergency department setting have been extensively studied. Several sets of guidelines have been derived. Two guidelines that are commonly cited include the Ottawa knee rules [4] and the Pittsburgh decision rules [5]. In a direct comparison, the latter were slightly more sensitive and moderately more specific for detection of a fracture [6]. The Pittsburgh rules call for radiographs in patients who have sustained blunt trauma or a fall and are (1) unable to walk four weight-bearing steps or (2) older than 50 years or younger than 12 years. Bauer and colleagues [7] added to the criteria the presence of effusion or ecchymosis on physical examination. The clinical experience of the author suggests that the office internist would be well served by obtaining knee radiographs in patients who have a history of blunt trauma or twisting injury and one of the following: age over 50 years, inability to walk four steps comfortably, and knee effusion or ecchymosis on physical examination.

Knee fractures

Tibial plateau, proximal fibula, and patella fractures may present primarily to the primary care physician's office. Tibial plateau fractures in the office setting may be subtle. Lateral plateau fractures are more common and the result of valgus stress and abduction forces. Medial plateau fractures are the result of varus stress and adduction forces. Physical examination commonly reveals effusion from hemarthrosis and decreased range of motion. Associated ligamentous injuries may be present. Neurovascular examination is important because of the proximity of the popliteal artery to the plateau. The diagnosis may be made with plain radiographs, but oblique views may be necessary to diagnose nondisplaced or minimally displaced fractures. In the setting of strong clinical suspicion but negative plain radiographs, CT or MRI is indicated. When fracture displacement is present, urgent orthopedic consultation should be initiated.

Patellar fractures are typically the result of a fall or direct blow. Clinical findings include pain, tenderness, and ecchymosis. Inability to extend the leg suggests disruption of the extensor mechanism. Proximal fibula fractures present with pain associated with walking following a direct blow to the leg. Because the peroneal nerve surrounds the fibular neck, a complete neurovascular examination is important. Foot drop may be seen with peroneal nerve injury.

The acute treatment of all office knee fractures is similar. Patients should be made non–weight bearing and treated with analgesics. Initial immobilization is indicated. A compressive dressing may provide symptomatic relief. Ice and elevation minimize swelling. Patients should be advised of warning signs of compartment syndrome. Consultation with an orthopedic surgeon for follow-up evaluation is appropriate.

Ligamentous injuries

The four major knee ligaments are the anterior cruciate ligament (ACL), posterior cruciate ligament (PCL), medial collateral ligament (MCL), and lateral collateral ligament (LCL) (see Fig. 1). The American Medical Association provides a clinically useful system for grading ligamentous injuries [8]. Grade I injuries describe ligamentous stretching without loss of integrity. This grade is assigned to patients in whom tenderness but no laxity is noted on stress examination. Grade II injuries indicate a partial tear. The physical examination correlate is laxity on stress examination with a firm endpoint. Grade III injuries are those with complete disruption of the ligament. Physical examination reveals laxity and no firm endpoint.

Plain radiographs in patients who have suspected ligamentous injuries include the anteroposterior, lateral, intercondylar notch, and sunrise views.

Bony pathology accompanying ligamentous injuries includes avulsion fractures from the site of attachment, osteochondral injuries, and loose bodies. MRI is a superb tool for the diagnosis of ligamentous injuries. It is highly sensitive in cases of complete ruptures and very useful for identifying associated or alternate diagnoses. The study is cost effective because it decreases the number of negative arthroscopies and unnecessary orthopedic referrals [3].

Valgus and varus stress injuries are the usual mechanisms for injuries to the MCL and LCL, respectively. Isolated injuries to these ligaments are usually treated conservatively regardless of grade [9]. Goals of therapy are pain control, restoration of range of motion, and protection from further injury. Strategies include nonsteroidal anti-inflammatory drugs (NSAIDs), ice, knee immobilization, and crutches for partial or non–weight bearing. Physical therapy may improve range of motion.

The ACL is the primary knee stabilizer. ACL rupture is a common serious injury allowing displacement of the tibia on the femur. Sporting injuries, particularly skiing and football, are common precipitants. Mechanisms of injury include hyperextension or valgus stress accompanied by external rotation of the tibia. Acute hemarthrosis frequently accompanies this injury and warrants early MRI and orthopedic referral [9].

The PCL is the strongest of the knee ligaments and less commonly injured in sporting accidents. Major trauma such as dashboard injury is a more common mechanism. Isolated PCL rupture is rare. Concurrent injuries to posterolateral structures, the MCL, or the ACL are frequently present [3].

Meniscal injuries

The medial and lateral menisci are C-shaped fibrocartilaginous structures that act as shock absorbers between the tibia and femur. Meniscal injuries are the most common knee injuries. History and physical examination are quite sensitive and specific for identification of meniscal injury. Mechanisms include twisting motions or rapid flexion/extension maneuvers while bearing weight. Degenerative disease may cause injury alone or in conjunction with acute injury. Historical features that suggest meniscal injury are locking, giving away, joint line pain, and swelling. Knee effusions that accompany meniscal injuries occur over 12 to 24 hours in contrast to the immediate swelling seen with ACL tears. Physical examination may reveal a locked knee, joint effusion, or tenderness along the joint line. McMurray's test and the Apley compression test are often positive [3,9].

Plain radiographs reveal no specific findings in isolated meniscal injuries. MRI is the confirmatory imaging study of choice. The accuracy for meniscal tear detection exceeds 90% [10]. Arthroscopy is the "gold standard" for diagnosis.

An acutely locked knee warrants manipulation to reduce the torn meniscus. Office strategy begins with intra-articular injection of local anesthetic. The leg should be allowed to hang off the bed in 90° degrees of flexion.

Gentle rotation generally reduces the fragment. Initial treatment is otherwise conservative; compression wrap, ice, elevation, analgesics, and crutches as needed constitute appropriate care [9]. Surgical excision of an unstable meniscal fragment is definitive orthopedic treatment [11].

Extensor mechanism rupture

The extensor mechanism includes the quadriceps muscles, quadriceps tendon, patella, and patellar tendon (Fig. 2). Injury resulting in interruption can occur anywhere along the continuum. A direct blow such as a fall on the patella is a direct mechanism of injury. Forced flexion of an extended knee constitutes an indirect mechanism. Pertinent historical features are sudden pain associated with a pop or tear. Hemarthrosis usually accompanies patellar tendon rupture [12]. The hallmark of the physical examination is inability to fully extend the knee and hold it up against gravity. The appropriate examination is to ask the patient to lie supine on a table and lift the extended leg. A palpable defect overlying the quadriceps or patellar

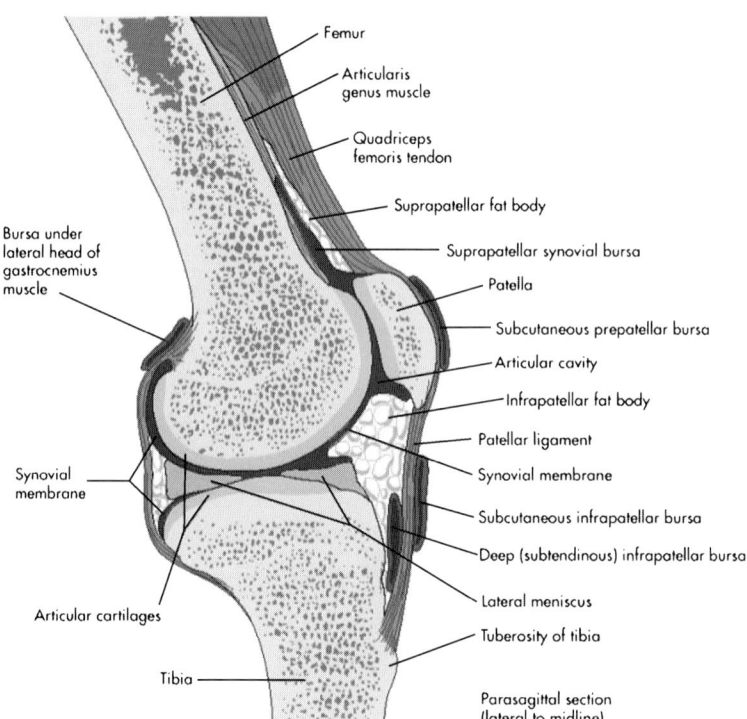

Fig. 2. Anatomy of the extensor mechanism of the knee. (*From* Marx JA, Hockberger RS, Walls RM, editors. Rosen's emergency medicine: concepts and clinical practice. 5th edition. St. Louis (MO): Mosby; 2002. p. 685. Copyright © 2002 Mosby, Inc.; with permission.)

tendon is present in either of these injuries. Patients who have patellar fractures have exquisite tenderness over the patella. It is important to note that patients who have incomplete tears may retain the ability to extend the leg.

Plain radiographs are indicated in extensor mechanism injuries. Patella fractures may be diagnosed. In the absence of fracture, patellar displacement is suggestive of tendon rupture. Patella baja is the term for inferior displacement seen with quadriceps tendon rupture, and patella alta is seen with the superior patellar displacement of patellar tendon rupture [9,13]. MRI or ultrasound are indicated in suspected partial tendon ruptures.

Knee immobilization in extension is the appropriate initial intervention for extensor mechanism injuries. Crutches, rest, ice, and elevation constitute adjunctive treatment. Early orthopedic consultation is appropriate. Most patients who have complete extensor mechanism rupture require surgical correction [9,12].

Overuse injuries

Gradual onset of pain in a patient who has a history of repetitive stress to the knee is characteristic of an overuse syndrome. Pain location may be medial, lateral, or peripatellar. Patients usually give a history of participation in sports or athletic training [3]. Factors such as poor training technique or improper shoes contribute to overuse injuries. The physiologic insult occurs when tissue repair is overcome by repetitive injury. Microtrauma precipitates soft tissue inflammation.

Patellofemoral syndrome

Patellofemoral pain syndrome (PFS) (also called chondromalacia patellae) is a common condition in young women with chronic anterior knee pain. Patients are often athletic and give histories of weight-bearing activities. Jogging, volleyball, and basketball are commonly associated with PFS. Typically, the discomfort is worsened by prolonged sitting, climbing stairs, and kneeling. On physical examination, patients may demonstrate an antalgic gait. A slight effusion may be present. When testing range of motion, crepitus is commonly found. Palpating the anterior patella reproduces the patient's pain, particularly along the inferior pole. Knee examination should include palpation of the superior and inferior patellar facets and compression testing for apprehension to medial or lateral subluxation [14]. Not all patients who have PFS require diagnostic imaging. Plain radiographs add little to the evaluation but may rule out other conditions such as arthritis. CT and MRI are not indicated unless the patient does not respond to conservative treatment [15].

The specific lesion causing PFS is unclear. Arthroscopic examination does not reveal anatomic abnormalities. Patellofemoral maltracking, subchondral bone pathology, increased intraosseous pressure, and early articular degeneration are among current etiologic theories [11].

Treatment of PFS is conservative and includes several modalities. Physical therapy focuses on quadriceps strengthening and stretching. Ice and NSAIDS are useful for pain control and reduction of inflammation. Activity modification, with particular focus on those activities known to precipitate PFS, is important. Brace support of the patellofemoral mechanism may be employed. Pain reduction and functional improvement are the therapeutic goals. Some cases of PFS prove refractory to these regimens and become chronic cases. Referral to an orthopedic surgeon is appropriate; however, arthroscopy may worsen the patient's condition [3,11].

Patellar tendonopathy

Athletes involved in sports associated with jumping or repeated stress to the extensor mechanism of the knee are at risk for development of patellar tendinopathy. Commonly called "jumper's knee," the condition is frequently diagnosed in basketball and volleyball players but may be seen in athletes participating in other sports including those without significant jumping. Early in the syndrome, patients note a dull aching sensation in the anterior knee following strenuous activity. Pain may accompany descending stairs and prolonged sitting. If unaddressed, pain may occur during athletic activity and degrade performance.

The main physical finding in patients who have patellar tendinopathy is tenderness over the patellar tendon, most frequently noted at the superior aspect of the tendon and inferior pole of the patella. Pain is affected by the position of the knee. Flexing the knee to 90° increases tension over the tendon; tenderness is decreased on examination. The most reliable position for eliciting tenderness and confirming the diagnosis is full extension. Placing pressure on the superior pole of the patella elevates the inferior pole and allows the examiner to palpate the origin of the patellar tendon [16].

A four-level clinical grading scale for patellar tendinopathy was developed by Blazina and colleagues [17] and is useful in the office setting. In the first stage, patients note pain only after athletic activity. In the second stage, pain occurs during activity but performance is not adversely affected. Deterioration of athletic performance heralds stage 3 and pain is prolonged. Blazina stage 4 is reached when the patellar tendon ruptures. Biedert [18] inserted a stage characterized by partial tendon rupture between Blazina stages 3 and 4.

The main consideration in the differential diagnosis of patellar tendinopathy is PFS. In some patients, the conditions coexist. Other entities that must be differentiated include meniscal tears and cartilage degeneration [16]. Imaging is indicated when the diagnosis is unclear. The two most useful modalities are ultrasonography and MRI. The former identifies tendon lesions by decreased echogenicity caused by disruption of collagen bundles. Tendon thickening, calcifications, and erosion of the patellar tip may be identified by ultrasound. MRI provides detailed images of the structures of the knee including the patellar tendon. Tendinopathy manifests a focal signal increase and thickening of the tendon [16]. Partial tears within the tendon are frequently identified [19].

The pathophysiology of patellar tendinopathy is tendinosis, a degenerative condition; it is to be distinguished from tendonitis, an inflammatory condition. Tendinosis is caused by progressive tissue degeneration and the failure of regeneration. Inflammatory cells are not found. The pathologic tendon develops a yellow-brown disorganized appearance that is distinctly different from the healthy white, organized, and glistening appearance of a normal tendon [16].

The initial approach to patellar tendinopathy is conservative. Relative rest, including two components, is recommended. The first component is cessation of jumping activities or other maneuvers causing excessive patellar loading. Temporarily decreasing total training hours is the second. Strengthening exercises and proper stretching are appropriate. Ice, massage, and NSAIDs are ancillary treatment modalities. Because of the absence of inflammation in the pathophysiology of patellar tendinopathy, the role of NSAIDS and corticosteroid injections is debated. Some studies show pain relief with NSAIDs but the actual effect on tendon healing is unclear [20]. Because inflammatory pathways may be involved in the pathogenesis, NSAIDs are still recommended. The slow metabolic rate of tendon tissue delays the progress of conservative treatment. Surgery should not be considered until at least 6 months of a well-supervised conservative program has failed. Multiple surgical approaches exist, with no consensus as to the most optimal. One review found that 15% to 25% of patients had persistent or recurrent pain following surgery for patellar tendinopathy [13].

Iliotibial band friction syndrome

Lateral knee pain in an active patient is characteristic of iliotibial band friction syndrome (ITBFS). The syndrome accounts for approximately 14% of overuse injuries of the knee [21]. Typical patients include long distance runners, cyclists, skiers, and military personnel. Historical features include pain or burning sensation over the lateral knee that is exacerbated by running. In early cases of ITBFS, symptoms subside after running; later in the syndrome, symptoms persist during normal activities.

The defining feature of the physical examination of patients who have ITBFS is marked point tenderness over the lateral femoral epicondyle. Joint effusion is not precipitated by the syndrome. Palpation of the iliotibial band may elicit a rubbing or snapping sensation. The compression test (Noble's test) is performed with the knee flexed to 90°. The examiner palpates the affected epicondyle and gradually extends the knee. The test is positive for ITBFS if the patient's symptoms are reproduced at 30° of flexion [22].

The diagnosis of ITBFS is clinical in patients who have characteristic historical and physical features [23]. Plain radiographs reveal no characteristic findings and are only of value in ruling out other pathology. MRI reveals thickening of the iliotibital band. Surrounding fluid, distinct from a joint effusion, may be noted superficially and deep to the band [19]. MRI is indicated in patients in whom the diagnosis is in question or preoperatively in patients considered for surgery [22].

Management of ITBFS is initially conservative. First-line treatment includes a short period of abstinence from precipitating athletic activities. At the time of resumption, an aggressive stretching program should be initiated. The goal of stretching is reduction of the compressive force between the lateral epicondyle and the iliotibial band. Adjunctive measures include NSAIDs, ice, and gluteus strengthening exercises. The next line of therapy consists of physical therapy referral, orthotics in patients who have excessive foot pronation, and corticosteroid injection into the bursa [11]. Surgery should be considered a last resort and only after a minimum of 6 months of nonoperative management. Surgical intervention consists of transection of the posterior portion of the band where it passes over the femoral epicondyle and excision of the bursa. One study documented that 84.4% of patients had good or excellent results following surgery and that 75.6% of patients retrospectively stated they would have the surgery again [24].

Medial knee overuse syndromes

Medial plica syndrome may develop in runners. The plica, a normal finding in most people, is a joint synovium redundancy located along the midmedial retinaculum that becomes inflamed with overuse. Physical examination is remarkable for tenderness over the plica. In patients who have marked hypertrophy, a mobile and nodular band is appreciated anterior to the medial joint line. No joint effusion accompanies the syndrome [11,14]. The diagnosis is clinical. No characteristic findings are identified on plain films or bone scans. MRI may identify a hypertrophied plica. Like other overuse syndromes, initial management includes NSAIDs, ice, and physical therapy. Orthopedic referral and arthroscopic resection should be considered after 6 months of failed conservative treatment.

The other main overuse entity in the differential diagnosis for medial knee pain is pes anserine bursitis. The pes anserine bursa is formed by the tendinous insertions of the sartorius, gracilus, and semitendinosus muscles. The bursa is located along the anteromedial aspect of the proximal tibia distal to the joint line and posterior to the MCL. Patients present with pain and tenderness directly over the bursa. There is no joint effusion but swelling of the bursa may be identified. Flexion, extension, and valgus stress testing reproduce the pain. Potential etiologies include overuse and direct trauma [14]. Pes anserine bursitis is uncommon and may be confused with medial collateral ligaments strain or internal knee derangement. MRI is the diagnostic study of choice, revealing a characteristic fluid collection beneath the tendons of the pes anserinus in the absence of other knee structure abnormalities [25]. Treatment includes NSAIDs, ice, relative rest, and compression [26].

Ankle injuries

Injuries to the foot and ankle are the most common injuries suffered by athletes (Figs. 3–5) [27]. History and physical examination augmented by appropriate imaging identifies the correct diagnosis in most injuries. The immediate development of marked swelling and severe pain suggest fracture, ligamentous disruption, or tendon rupture. The patient's recall of a "pop" is consistent with any of these injuries. An inversion injury is the most common mechanism for sprain of the lateral ligaments but may also precipitate a fifth metatarsal fracture.

Physical examination of the patient who has an ankle injury should begin with a screening assessment of the knee to exclude associated injury, particularly fracture of the proximal fibula. Ankle inspection identifies deformity, ecchymosis, and edema. Palpation of bony structures includes the medial and lateral malleoli, the entire length of the tibia and fibula, tibial plafond, the talus, the calcaneus, and the base of the fifth metatarsal. Ligamentous structures requiring palpation are the LCL and the syndesmotic ligaments. The Achilles and peroneal tendons should be palpated and assessed for integrity. When the examination is negative for marked swelling, ecchymosis, or bony tenderness, assessing the ability to ambulate is appropriate. Stress testing of the ankle should be performed only when fracture is ruled out [28].

Routine radiographic imaging of the ankle includes anteroposterior, lateral, and 20° internal oblique (mortise) views. Foot imaging includes anteroposterior, lateral, and oblique views [29]. The Ottawa ankle rules [30,31] have been demonstrated to limit unnecessary ankle and foot imaging in

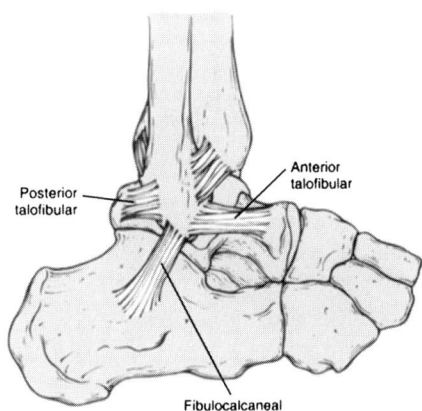

Fig. 3. Anatomy of the LCL. (*From* Browner. Skeletal trauma: basic science, management, and reconstruction. 3rd edition. Philadelphia: Elsevier; 2003. p. 2310. Copyright © 2003 Elsevier.)

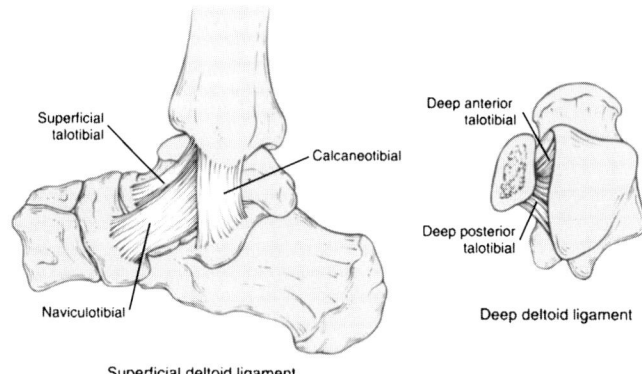

Fig. 4. Medial ankle ligaments. (*From* Browner. Skeletal trauma: basic science, management, and reconstruction. 3rd edition. Philadelphia: Elsevier; 2003. p. 2308. Copyright © 2003 Elsevier; with permission.)

emergency department patients while maintaining high sensitivity for detection of ankle and midfoot fractures [32]. The rules state that ankle radiographs are indicated when the patient has malleolar pain and any of the following:

- Tenderness at the posterior edge of the distal 6 cm or the tip of the lateral malleolus
- Tenderness at the posterior edge of the distal 6 cm or the tip of the medial malleolus
- Inability to bear four steps of weight immediately after the injury and at the time of physician evaluation

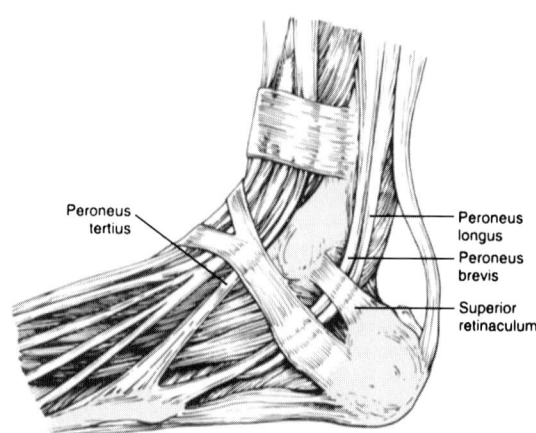

Fig. 5. Peroneus longus and brevis tendons. (*From* Browner. Skeletal trauma: basic science, management, and reconstruction. 3rd edition. Philadelphia: Elsevier; 2003. p. 2310. Copyright © 2003 Elsevier; with permission.)

Foot radiographs should be obtained when there is midfoot pain and any of the following:

- Navicular bone tenderness
- Tenderness at the base of the fifth metatarsal
- Inability to bear four steps of weight immediately after the injury and at the time of physician evaluation

The recommendations regarding foot radiography apply only to the midfoot region and to injuries covered by the Ottawa ankle rules. They are not general guidelines for imaging patients who have isolated foot injuries.

CT is not indicated for the initial evaluation of ankle or foot injuries. Because of its superior imaging of bones, CT may be used to diagnose subtle fractures in patients who have negative plain radiographs and in whom the physician maintains a high index of suspicion for fracture. MRI may be used for patients who have subacute or chronic complaints of ankle pain or to evaluate suspected tendon injuries [29].

Ankle fractures

It is unlikely that patients who have displaced or unstable bimalleolar or trimalleolar fractures will present to a primary care office. All such injuries require urgent orthopedic consultation, and these patients should be sent to an emergency department. Nondisplaced lateral malleolar fractures below the tibiotalar joint without associated medial ankle injury may be splinted in the office and referred to an orthopedist. All patients should be made non–weight bearing, fitted with crutches, and treated with rest, ice, and elevation. Because the fibula is not a weight-bearing bone, it can be managed nonoperatively.

Medial malleolar fractures are the result of eversion or external rotation. They are commonly associated with lateral or posterior malleolar fractures. A Maisonneuve fracture is the coexistence of a proximal fibular fracture with a medial malleolar fracture. All medial malleolar fractures require emergency orthopedic consultation.

Ankle sprains

Most ankle sprains are the result of inversion injuries and involve the LCL. These include the anterior talofibular ligament, the calcaneofibular ligament, and the posterior talofibular ligament (see Fig. 3). Two thirds of ankle sprains are isolated to the anterior talofibular ligament. Twenty percent of sprains involve the anterior talofibular ligament and calcaneofibular ligament. The medial or deltoid ligament is strong and thick (see Fig. 4); it is involved in fewer than 5% of sprains [28]. A very strong syndesmotic ligament attaches the distal tibia and fibula and maintains ankle mortice integrity. It is rarely sprained because of its great strength.

Patients who have ankle sprains usually maintain the ability to walk on the affected extremity. Those with third-degree sprains may give a history of a snap or pop. Physical examination reveals tenderness over the affected ligament. Injury to the syndesmotic ligament causes pain just above the ankle with compression of the tibia and fibula. A third-degree ankle sprain of the anterior talofibular ligament is characterized by a positive ankle drawer sign. The examiner cups one hand over the heel and pulls the foot anteriorly while the other hand provides countertraction over the front of the tibia. The sign is positive when movement of the foot is disproportionate to the unaffected side and a firm endpoint is absent. Acutely injured patients may be too tender to tolerate the drawer sign.

Subtle foot and ankle fractures often masquerade as ankle sprains. Nondisplaced talar dome fractures may not be evident on plain radiographs. When primary care physicians follow up patients diagnosed with ankle sprains who are not progressing as expected, this possibility should be considered. CT or MRI is indicated for further evaluation [33]. Fractures of the base of the fifth metatarsal appear similar to ankle sprains on clinical examination. Point tenderness in this region should prompt an order for a radiograph.

First- and second-degree sprains are appropriate for office management. Initial treatment is RICE therapy (rest, ice, compression, elevation) and crutches for non–weight bearing. Older patients may do better with a cane for minor injuries or a walker for more serious sprains. Analgesics are appropriate for pain. An elastic bandage is suitable for compression. Ankle immobilization devices such as air casts or stirrup splints assist with joint protection, particularly when the patient resumes ambulation. A second phase of treatment begins when the swelling and pain decrease and the patient can comfortably bear weight. Ankle strengthening exercises are appropriate at this stage. Research has shown that early weight bearing produces superior results to prolonged immobilization [34].

Tendon injuries

The Achilles tendon is the largest tendon in the body. It spans two joints and connects the gastrocnemius and soleus muscles of the calf to the calcaneus. A limited blood supply and high stress forces render the tendon vulnerable to injury. Men in the fourth decade who engage in jumping or sprinting sports are most at risk for tendon rupture. Historical clues to rupture are the feeling of a "snap" or "pop" following a jump or other sudden motion. Physical examination reveals edema and ecchymosis overlying the ruptured tendon. The patient has weakened or absent ability to plantarflex the foot. A gap in the Achilles tendon is often palpable. The Thompson test is diagnostic. This test is best performed by having the patient lie prone on the examining table with his or her feet hanging off the end. The examiner compresses the calf muscles. Absence of plantar flexion is consistent with a ruptured Achilles. Imaging is unnecessary unless the examination is equivocal. MRI or ultrasound is then indicated [27]. Patients should be splinted, given crutches for ambulation, and urgently referred to an orthopedist. Treatment options are surgery plus immobilization or immobilization alone. Athletes are most often treated surgically, with the goal of early return to sports [35].

Achilles tendonitis develops in about 10% of runners but is seen in other physically active persons. Patients complain of pain along the tendon or at its calcaneus insertion. Physical examination is positive for tenderness with palpation of the tendon or with active range of motion. Initial treatment is rest, ice, and NSAIDs. Other considerations are warming up and stretching before exercise and icing afterwards. Physical therapy referral for ultrasound and flexibility training is appropriate. Referral for possible surgical management is indicated if patients do not improve with 6 months of conservative management [35].

The peroneus longus and brevis muscles evert, pronate, and participate in plantar flexion of the foot. Their tendons run along the fibular groove behind the lateral malleolus and insert into the metatarsals (see Fig. 5). Dislocation or subluxation of the tendons occurs when there is injury to the superior peroneal retinaculum attachment to the fibula. Forced dorsiflexion is the most common mechanism of injury. Patients complain of pain and a snapping sensation in the posterolateral aspect of the ankle. Dislocated tendons may be palpable. Swelling and tenderness are typically seen on physical examination. Confusion with ankle sprains and resultant misdiagnosis are common. On physical examination, the patient may be unable to evert the ankle while dorsiflexed, which distinguishes peroneal tendon injury from a lateral ankle sprain. The tendons may sublux with dorsiflexion or with circular rolling of the foot. All patients who have peroneal tendon injuries require orthopedic referral. Treatment is controversial but usually requires surgery [36].

Shoulder injuries

The shoulder is an elegant anatomic structure that is composed of three joints: the glenohumeral, the acromioclavicular, and the sternoclavicular (Fig. 6). The design maximizes range of motion and flexibility at the expense of stability. The shallow osseous coverage of the glenoid fossa allows freedom of humeral movement but relies on nonbony structures including the joint capsule, ligaments, and muscles for support. The complexities of the shoulder design increase its susceptibility to dislocation, chronic instability, and degenerative changes.

Historical features of importance in patients who have shoulder trauma are mechanism of injury, pain location, motion limitation, precipitating and alleviating factors, and presence or absence of neurologic symptoms. In patients who do not have an obvious precipitating injury, rapidity of

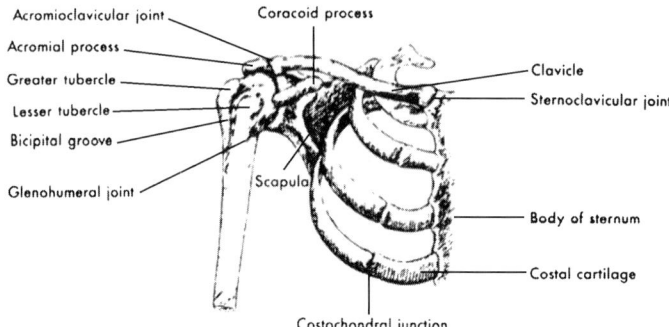

Fig. 6. Shoulder. (*From* In: Marx JA, Hockberger RS, Walls RM, editors. Rosen's emergency medicine: concepts and clinical practice. 5th edition. St. Louis (MO): Mosby; 2002. p. 577. Copyright © 2002 Mosby Inc.; with permission.)

onset should be determined. Patient factors such as age, activity level, habitus, occupation, and emotional state are important when evaluating shoulder pain [37]. Pathologic processes of many etiologies cause radiating pain to the shoulder. Consideration must be given to cervical spine, vascular, cardiac, pulmonary, and gastrointestinal diseases in patients whose chief complaint is shoulder pain.

Physical examination begins with inspection. Swelling, ecchymosis, symmetry with the unaffected shoulder, atrophy, muscle tone, fasciculations, and abnormal posturing should be noted. Active range of motion including flexion, extension, abduction, adduction, internal rotation, and external rotation should be assessed. Palpation should cover examinations of the sternoclavicular and acromioclavicular joints, scapula, clavicle, and humerus. The rotator cuff muscles and others making up the shoulder joint (latisimus dorsi, teres major, pectoralis major and minor, deltoid) should be palpated (Fig. 7). A thorough neurovascular examination of the upper extremity completes the examination.

Plain radiographs should be ordered in patients evaluated for traumatic injuries. Trauma views include a true anteroposterior, transscapular lateral, and axillary [38]. When obtaining radiographs in patients who have pain but no history of trauma, standard views are anteroposterior with the beam centered on the coracoid process; internal and external rotation views are obtained [37]. MRI is an outstanding study for diagnosing pathology of the soft tissues of the shoulder [39].

Shoulder fractures

Fractures of the clavicle and proximal humerus may present to the outpatient physician office as primary injuries or for follow-up care. Scapular fractures are uncommon and require considerable force such as that sustained from a high-speed vehicular accident or a fall from height [38].

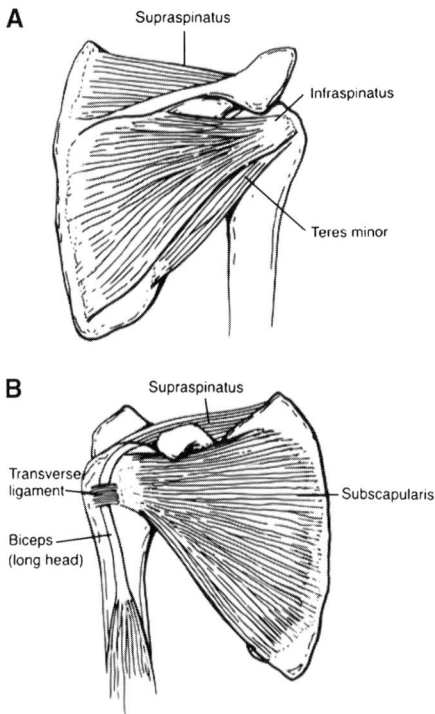

Fig. 7. Rotator cuff anatomy: (*A*) posterior and (*B*) anterior views. (*From* DeLee J, Drez D, editors. DeLee and Drez's orthopaedics sports medicine: principles and practice. 2nd edition. Philadelphia: Elsevier; 2003. p. 1066. Copyright © 2003 Elsevier; with permission.)

They are unlikely to be treated in the office setting. Clavicular fractures require a careful neurovascular examination because of the proximity to the brachial plexus and subclavian vessels. Assuming the absence of neurovascular injury, pneumothorax, or other major injury, patients can be initially managed with a sling, ice, and analgesia. A figure-eight bandage may be used; however, no evidence supports its efficacy in reduction of the clavicular fracture [40]. Fractures of the middle third of the clavicle with greater than 20 mm of displacement have a high incidence of nonunion and unsatisfactory results with conservative management [41]. These injuries should be referred to an orthopedist for follow-up care. In the absence of significant displacement, most patients recover with a satisfactory outcome following conservative treatment from a primary care physician.

Proximal humerus fractures are common injuries in the elderly population. Unlike young patients who are more likely to dislocate the shoulder with trauma, elderly patients fracture. Nordqvist and Petersson [42] reported 67 years as the mean age of patients who sustain these injuries. Osteoporosis weakens the bone and predisposes it to fracture. Eighty-five percent of proximal humerus fractures are minimally displaced and may be managed with a sling and swathe, ice, and analgesia. Some evidence suggests that patients benefit from physical therapy as early as 1 week post injury [43]. The Neer classification system defines significant displacement as angulation exceeding 45° or fracture fragments separated by more than 1 cm [44]. Patients who have humeral fractures may require surgical intervention and should be referred to an orthopedist.

Separation of the coracoacromial junction is a common injury in athletic young men. The usual mechanism is a fall or direct blow to the shoulder. The Tossy and Allman classification divides the injuries into types I, II, and III based on the degree of ligamentous disruption. Regardless of type, most patients are well served by conservative treatment with a sling, ice, and analgesia. Range-of-motion exercises and shoulder strengthening should be initiated when pain subsides; in most cases, this occurs within 1 to 3 weeks [45]. Type III injuries (complete ligamentous disruption) have no better outcomes when managed operatively compared with conservative treatment [46].

Painful shoulder syndromes

A subacute syndrome of shoulder pain commonly presenting to the office is referred to by multiple names: supraspinatus tendonitis, rotator cuff tendonitis, calcific tendonitis, subacromial bursitis, subdeltoid bursitis, impingement syndrome, and painful arc syndrome, among others [37]. The condition is part of a pathologic continuum, the endpoint of which is rupture of the rotator cuff [38] (see Fig. 7). Rotator cuff tendonitis, the lesion responsible for this syndrome, is most likely a combination of inflammation, hypovascularity, degeneration, and impingement. Some occupations, particularly those that require recurrent overhead activity, accelerate the process. Neer classifies the continuum into three stages [47]. In the first, patients note a dull ache after activity. Tenderness is found over the acromion process and the supraspinatus. Stage 2 is heralded by night pain thought to be the result of bursal inflammation and subsequent adhesions. Physical findings are the same as the first stage. Terms such as adhesive capsulitis, adhesive bursitis, and frozen shoulder describe stage 2 of the rotator cuff syndrome [37].

Rotator cuff rupture, stage 3 of the syndrome, may be an acute injury (10%) characterized by forced abduction or chronic tear (90%) presenting in a subacute fashion. Arm weakness heralds stage 3. Inability to abduct the arm is the primary physical finding. Plain radiographs may reveal indirect findings of rotator cuff rupture, but MRI will confirm the diagnosis [38].

Management of stages I and II of rotator cuff tendonitis is rest, gradual introduction of strengthening exercises, and NSAIDs. Immobilization should be avoided. Subacromial injections of lidocaine and corticosteroids may be efficacious in patients who have stage II disease. Patients who have rotator cuff tears should be immobilized in a sling, given analgesics for pain, and expeditiously referred to an orthopedist [37,38]. Small tears may respond to conservative management and physical therapy. Large lesions often require surgical repair [40].

Elbow injuries

The elbow is a hinge joint that exchanges mobility for stability. Three bones articulate to form the joint: the humerus tapering into medial and lateral condyles, the radius, and the ulna. The trochlea, the articular surface of the medial condyle, articulates with the olecranon and coronoid processes of the ulna to form the hinge joint. The capitellum, the articular surface of the lateral condyle, articulates with the radius; the radial head articulates with the radial notch of the ulna. Four clinically important ligaments provide support to the elbow: the radial collateral ligament, the ulnar collateral ligament, the annular ligament, and the anterior capsule (Fig. 8). Three bursae surround the elbow; the most clinically significant is the olecranon bursa located posterior to the olecranon process [48].

Historical features of importance in patients who have elbow injuries are mechanism of injury and symptoms of neurovascular injury distal to the elbow. Patients presenting subacutely with elbow pain should be questioned

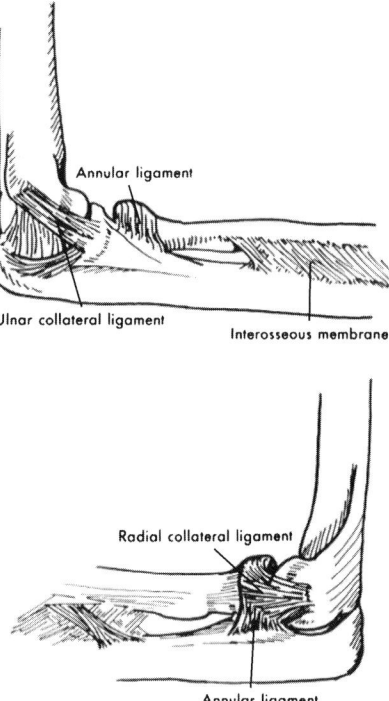

Fig. 8. Elbow anatomy. (*From* Marx JA, Hockberger RS, Walls RM, editors. Rosen's emergency medicine: concepts and clinical practice. 5th edition. St. Louis (MO): Mosby; 2002. p. 556. Copyright © 2002 Mosby, Inc.; with permission.)

about provocative and alleviating activities. Physical examination begins with inspection for deformity, ecchymosis, and edema. Elbow palpation should detect tenderness, with specific attention to the radial head. Acutely injured patients require a thorough neurovascular assessment with the goal of detecting signs of compartment syndrome (see Box 1). Early indicators are pain out of proportion to examination and severe pain with passive finger extension. These findings should prompt emergent orthopedic consultation. Range of motion should be assessed in patients who do not have evidence of serious injury. Normal flexion-extension is from 0° to 150° with the forearm supinated; normal pronation-supination is 90° with the elbow held in 90° of flexion [49].

Radiographic imaging of the injured elbow begins with plain radiographs. Most fractures are diagnosed with this modality. For patients who have persistent symptoms and negative plain films, MRI is the next appropriate study. It is an excellent modality for identification of osteochondral injuries; soft tissue structures such as ligaments, tendons, and cartilage are well visualized with MRI. Ultrasound imaging is useful in elbow evaluation because of the superficial nature of the elbow soft tissue structures. It is excellent for identifying and aspirating joint fluid; evaluation of supporting tendons and ligaments and limited imaging of articular cartilage may also be done [50].

Elbow fractures

Initial management of elbow fractures depends on the clinical presentation. Fractures that are displaced, unstable, or associated with neurovascular injury should be urgently referred to an orthopedic surgeon. Nondisplaced isolated injuries may be placed in a posterior elbow splint and sling and treated with ice and analgesics. Although most of these injuries should be referred to an orthopedist, this referral may occur in a less urgent time frame.

Radial head fractures are common injuries that may initially present to the outpatient setting. The usual mechanism is a fall on the outstretched hand. The Mason classification divides radial head fractures into four types: type I are nondisplaced, type II are displaced, type III are comminuted, and type IV are associated with a dislocation [51]. Ligamentous injuries may accompany radial head fractures; these include the MCL, LCL, or interosseous ligament joining the distal radius and ulna. Physical examination is positive for pain with flexion and extension and radial head tenderness. An effusion is usually present. Type I injuries are managed with a posterior elbow splint for 5 to 7 days followed by early range-of-motion exercises. Joint aspiration and intra-articular injection of local anesthesia relieves pain and assists with early range of motion [52]. Types II through IV should be referred to an orthopedist. Some type II injuries may be managed conservatively, but surgical intervention might be necessary.

Fractures involving the condyle should be referred to orthopedic surgeons. Intercondylar fractures are intra-articular and frequently difficult to manage. Transcondylar fractures, although not intra-articular, are also difficult because the distal fragment is small and patients are at high risk for loss of range of motion [53]. Olecranon fractures are intra-articular by definition and should be managed by orthopedists. Unless completely stable and nondisplaced, open reduction and internal fixation are usually necessary [52].

Tendon ruptures

Rupture of the distal biceps tendon is an injury that occurs in the dominant arm of male patients and is exceedingly rare in female patients. Athletes such as weightlifters and rugby players are at particular risk. The usual mechanism of injury is a rapidly applied load with the elbow flexed. Patients frequently feel a "pop" accompanied by sharp pain. Physical examination is positive for tenderness and swelling over the distal biceps. A tendinous defect is present distally, creating the "Popeye sign." Weakness with supination and elbow flexion occur. In complete ruptures, imaging is rarely necessary. Ultrasound and MRI may be helpful in diagnosing cases of incomplete rupture. Definitive treatment is surgical. Triceps tendon rupture is an extremely rare injury. Falling on the outstretched hand is a common mechanism. Physical examination reveals tenderness, swelling, and ecchymosis along the posterior elbow and the absence of extension on range-of-motion testing. The diagnosis is clinical, but plain radiographs are helpful in ruling out other diagnoses. Complete ruptures require surgical management [54].

Epicondylitis

Epicondylitis is a very common cause of subacute elbow pain. It is an overuse syndrome; the pathology is a tendinopathy rather than tendonitis. Histologic examination reveals angiofibroblastic hyperplasia without the presence of inflammatory cells. Lateral epicondylitis, or "tennis elbow," accounts for most cases. Tendons of the extensor carpi radialis brevis and extensor digitorum communis are the affected structures. Medial epicondylitis is commonly known as "golfer's elbow" and is responsible for 10% to 20% of cases. Tendons of the pronator teres, flexor carpi radialis, and palmaris longus are most commonly affected [55]. Posterior epicondylitis, the least common elbow tendinopathy, involves the triceps tendon. The demographic profile of the typical patient who has epicondylitis is a physically active adult over age 35 years who aggressively works out at least three times per week for at least 30 minutes per session [56].

The characteristic early history of epicondylitis is elbow pain associated with activity. As the disease progresses, rest pain occurs. Tenderness is palpable over the affected epicondyle. Medial epicondylitis is exacerbated by forearm pronation and wrist flexion. Lateral epicondylitis is worsened by wrist extension against resistance and maximal wrist flexion [57]. The differential diagnosis for elbow pain includes nerve compression syndromes of the radial and nerves, ligamentous injuries, synovitis, and plica syndrome. A careful history, physical examination, and imaging should establish the correct diagnosis. Electromyography is indicated in patients who have neurologic symptoms suggestive of nerve compression syndromes [55,56].

Ninety-five percent of patients who have epicondylitis respond to conservative management. The goals of therapy are to reduce the stress to which the tissue is exposed and improve the quality of the patient's tissue. The first phase of treatment begins with temporary abstinence from the precipitating activity. Ice is recommended for 15 to 20 minutes three to four times per day. A 10- to 14-day course of an NSAID completes this phase. The second phase of therapy is rehabilitative. Physical therapy consultation may be very helpful. Stretching and strengthening exercises are begun. High-voltage electrical stimulation may be efficacious. A third phase has the goal of returning athletes to participation in sports. Counterforce bracing helps maintain muscle balance during exercise and improves pain control [58]. Orthopedic consultation is indicated for patients who fail a 3- to 6-month trial of conservative treatment [55,56].

Wrist injuries

The wrist is an anatomically complex structure with intricate biomechanics. The bony substrate is composed of eight carpal bones arranged in two rows of four, the distal radius and ulna, and the proximal aspect of the metacarpals (Fig. 9). Articulations within the wrist are the distal radioulnar

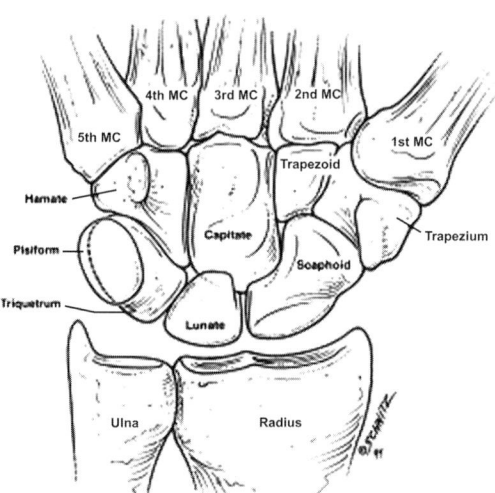

Fig. 9. Wrist bones. (Permission to reproduce this figure courtesy of Gary Schnitz, The Indiana Hand Center.)

joint, the radiocarpal joint, and the midcarpal joints. Flexor and extensor tendons course across the wrist along the volar and dorsal aspects, respectively, to provide fine motor coordination of the hand and phalanges [59]. Extrinsic and intrinsic ligaments stabilize the wrist (Fig. 10). The former connect the carpals to the radius and ulna proximally and the metacarpals distally; the latter connect and stabilize the carpals to one another. The ligamentous and tendonous structure allows flexion, extension, and radial and ulnar deviation of the wrist; pronation and supination occur at the distal radius and ulna [60].

The most important component of the history in a patient who has a wrist injury is the mechanism of injury. Certain injuries characteristically are the result of a fall on the outstretched hand and extremely unlikely in the absence of that mechanism. The site of maximum pain and tenderness is the second most important historical point.

Physical examination begins with inspection. The examiner should note the manner in which the wrist is held. Swelling, ecchymosis, erythema, and deformity should be noted. Comparison to the uninjured wrist is helpful in identifying pathologic changes. Range of motion should be tested in patients who do not have evidence of serious trauma. Palpation of the distal radius and ulna should be performed. The anatomic snuffbox is an important landmark. It is located along the radial aspect of the wrist and identified by having the patient radially deviate the hand and extend the thumb. The snuffbox is bordered by the abductor pollicis longus and extensor pollicis

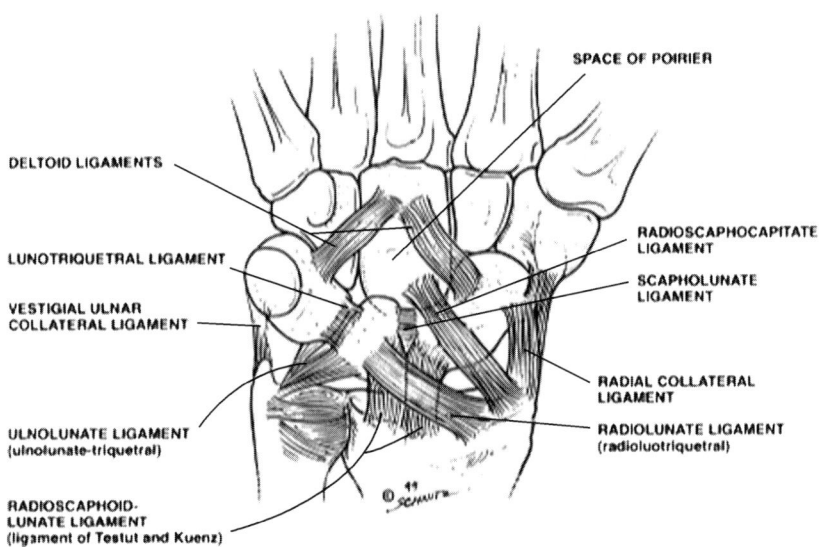

Fig. 10. Extrinsic and intrinsic wrist ligaments. (Permission to reproduce this figure courtesy of Gary Schnitz, The Indiana Hand Center.)

brevis tendons radially and the extensor pollicis longus tendon ulnarly. Palpating within the depression between the tendons identifies the scaphoid (or navicular). Lister's tubercle is the bony prominence palpable at the distal end of the radius. It provides a landmark for identification of the lunate and capitate. With the hand in neutral position, there is an indentation just proximal to the base of the third metacarpal and distal to Lister's tubercle. Palpation identifies the capitate. Flexing the wrist and palpating in the indentation identifies the lunate. Lister's tubercle, the lunate, the capitate, and the third metacarpal form a straight line in the uninjured wrist [48]. The pisiform is palpable along the ulnar aspect of the volar surface of the wrist just distal to the distal wrist crease. The neurovascular examination of the wrist and hand should be completed with documentation of presence of radial and ulnar arteries.

Radiographic evaluation of wrist injuries begins with plain films. Standard views are the posteroanterior, lateral, and oblique views. Additional views improve the sensitivity for diagnosing scaphoid fractures [61] or carpal ligament injuries. Because up to 15% of scaphoid fractures are missed with plain radiographs, bone scan may be used to make the diagnosis [62]. MRI is increasingly used when high clinical suspicion for injury persists in the face of negative plain radiographs. MRI has been shown to identify occult fractures in almost half of these patients and to identify significant soft tissue injuries in others [63,64]. Multidetector CT is an excellent modality for identification of occult carpal fractures in patients who have negative plain radiographs [65].

Wrist fractures

The distal radius is the most commonly fractured bone in the wrist. Three main fracture types occur with distinct mechanisms of injury: extension (Colles'), flexion (Smith's), and push-off (Hutchinson's and Barton's). More complex classifications are based on whether the fractures are intra- or extra-articular and involve injury to the ulna and the radioulnar joint. These classifications are beyond the scope of this article. CT or MRI may be necessary to define the complete extent of injury. All distal radius fractures should be referred to an orthopedist. Even when appropriately managed, the complication rate is high. Fractures that are extra-articular and nondisplaced without evidence of neurovascular injury may be placed in a sugar-tong splint with 15° of flexion and 15° of ulnar deviation and expeditiously referred. All others require initial treatment by the orthopedic specialist [48].

Scaphoid fracture is the most common fracture of the carpal bones. The tenuous blood supply is to the distal aspect of the bone. Undiagnosed fractures proximal to the blood supply leave patients with a high incidence of nonunion and avascular necrosis. The usual mechanism is forced hyperextension that occurs as the result of a fall on the outstretched hand. Patients present with pain and tenderness in the snuffbox. Because of the high incidence of negative films, such patients should be treated as fractured regardless of the results of plain radiographs. Diagnostic delay longer than 4 weeks or uncorrected displacement more than 1 mm is associated with adverse outcome. Open or closed reduction is indicated for displaced scaphoid fractures. Acute management of all scaphoid fractures is placement of a thumb spica splint, sling, ice, and analgesics. All of these fractures should be referred to an orthopedic surgeon for definitive care [66].

Lunate fractures represent less than 3% of all carpal fractures. The typical mechanism is a fall on the outstretched hand. Tenderness is present distal to Lister's tubercle with the wrist in flexion. Lunate fractures are concerning because of the risk of avascular necrosis known as Kienböck's disease, which occurs in approximately 20% of fractures. Radiographs demonstrate a sclerotic and ultimately collapsed lunate in late stages [67], which may be normal in early disease during which bone scan or MRI confirms the diagnosis. Kienböck's disease is commonly seen in athletes and thought to be an overuse syndrome [68]. Treatment is conservative in early stages; however, operative intervention is often necessary [67].

Fractures of the other carpals are far less common but do occur. Those that are isolated, nondisplaced, and not associated with ligamentous instability are usually managed with cast immobilization. Injuries complicated by displacement or instability often require surgical management and should be referred to an orthopedic surgeon [69].

Soft tissue wrist injuries

Wrist instability occurs with injury to the extrinsic or intrinsic wrist ligaments. When a partial injury occurs, the carpal bones remain normally aligned until a load is applied, at which time they collapse. This condition is referred to as dynamic instability. In severely damaged ligaments, bony alignment is abnormal on plain radiographs and is referred to as static instability [69]. Scapholunate instability is the most common ligamentous instability in the wrist. Severe pain is common. The Watson or scaphoid shift test is positive on physical examination. During this test, the physician places a thumb on the scaphoid tubercle while the patient's wrist is in ulnar deviation. The physician applies a palmarly directed force to the tubercle as the patient deviates the wrist in the radial direction. Severe pain indicates a positive test. Plain films may confirm the diagnosis; a gap between the scaphoid and the lunate exceeding 3 mm, the Terry Thomas sign, suggests scapholunate instability [59]. MRI may be indicated in patients who have negative plain films and high clinical suspicion. Open reduction and internal fixation is the definitive treatment [69]. Other instability syndromes occur with damage to the intrinsic ligaments far less commonly than scapholunate dissociation. Most can be treated conservatively with immobilization, analgesia, and activity modification, but those that do not respond require orthopedic evaluation.

Summary

Orthopedic injuries are common reasons for visits to primary care physicians. Careful history and physical examination with intelligent use of imaging technology will arrive at the correct diagnosis in most patients. Many conditions may be definitively managed by the office internist. Others may be initially stabilized and referred to orthopedic surgeons for definitive care. Nondisplaced fractures, tendon injuries, sprains, and overuse syndromes are entities within the purview of the primary care physician. Familiarity and confidence with diagnosis and management of these conditions in the office is optimal for the care of the adult patient.

References

[1] Amadio PC, Gabriel SE, Yawn BP, et al. Short-term outcomes of acute knee injuries: does the provider make a difference? Arthritis Rheum 2002;47:361–5.
[2] Calmbach WL, Hutchens M. Evaluation of patients presenting with knee pain. Part I: history, physical examination, radiographs, and laboratory tests. Am Fam Physician 2003; 68:907–12.
[3] Antosia R, Lyn E. Knee and lower leg. In: Marx J, Hockberger R, Walls R, editors. Rosen's emergency medicine: concepts and clinical practice. 5th edition. St. Louis (MO): Mosby; 2002. p. 674–97.
[4] Stiell IG, Greenberg GH, Wells GA, et al. Derivation of a decision rule for the use of radiography in acute knee injuries. Ann Emerg Med 1995;26:405–13.
[5] Seaberg DC, Jackson R. Clinical decision rule for knee radiographs. Am J Emerg Med 1994; 12:541–3.
[6] Seaberg DC, Yealy DM, Lukens T, et al. Multicenter comparison of two clinical decision rules for the use of radiography in acute, high-risk knee injuries. Ann Emerg Med 1998; 32:8–13.
[7] Bauer SJ, Hollander JE, Fuchs SH, et al. A clinical decision rule in the evaluation of acute knee injuries. J Emerg Med 1995;13:611–5.
[8] American Medical Association. Standard nomenclature of athletic injuries. Committee on the Medical Aspect of Sports. Chicago: American Medical Association; 1968.
[9] Perryman JR, Hershman EB. The acute management of soft tissue injuries of the knee. Orthop Clin North Am 2002;33:575–85.
[10] Anderson MW. MR imaging of the meniscus. Radiol Clin North Am 2002;40:1081–94.
[11] Kaeding C, Tomczak RL. Running injuries about the knee. Clin Podiatr Med Surg 2001;18: 307–18.
[12] Maffulli N, Wong J. Rupture of the Achilles and patellar tendons. Clin Sports Med 2003;22: 761–76.
[13] Coleman BD, Khan KM, Maffulli N, et al. Studies of surgical outcome after patellar tendinopathy: clinical significance of methodological deficiencies and guidelines for future studies. Victorian Institute of Sport Tendon Study Group. Scand J Med Sci Sports 2000;10:2–11.
[14] Calmbach WL, Hutchens M. Evaluation of patients presenting with knee pain. Part II: differential diagnosis. Am Fam Physician 2003;68:917–22.
[15] Taunton JE, Wilkinson M. Rheumatology: 14. Diagnosis and management of anterior knee pain. CMAJ 2001;164:1595–601.
[16] Warden SJ, Brukner P. Patellar tendinopathy. Clin Sports Med 2003;22:743–59.
[17] Blazina ME, Kerlan RK, Jobe FW, et al. Jumper's knee. Orthop Clin North Am 1973;4: 665–78.

[18] Biedert R. [Knee injuries in jogging.]. Schweiz Z Sportmed 1988;36:11–20.
[19] Carrino JA, Schweitzer ME. Imaging of sports-related knee injuries. Radiol Clin North Am 2002;40:181–202.
[20] Almekinders LC, Temple JD. Etiology, diagnosis, and treatment of tendonitis: an analysis of the literature. Med Sci Sports Exerc 1998;30:1183–90.
[21] Newell S, Bramwell S. Overuse injuries to the knee in runners. Phys Sportsmed 1984;12:81–6.
[22] Panni AS, Biedert RM, Maffulli N, et al. Overuse injuries of the extensor mechanism in athletes. Clin Sports Med 2002;21:483–98.
[23] Kirk KL, Kuklo T, Klemme W. Iliotibial band friction syndrome. Orthopedics 2000;23: 1209–14 [discussion: 1205–14; quiz 1207–16].
[24] Drogset JO, Rossvoll I, Grontvedt T. Surgical treatment of iliotibial band friction syndrome. A retrospective study of 45 patients. Scand J Med Sci Sports 1999;9:296–8.
[25] Forbes JR, Helms CA, Janzen DL. Acute pes anserine bursitis: MR imaging. Radiology 1995;194:525–7.
[26] Butcher JD, Salzman KL, Lillegard WA. Lower extremity bursitis. Am Fam Physician 1996; 53:2317–24.
[27] Title CI, Katchis SD. Traumatic foot and ankle injuries in the athlete. Orthop Clin North Am 2002;33:587–98.
[28] Ho K, Abu-Laban RB. Ankle and foot. In: Marx J, Hockberger R, Walls R, editors. Rosen's emergency medicine: concepts and clinical practice. 5th edition. St. Louis (MO): Mosby; 2002. p. 706–37.
[29] Dunfee WR, Dalinka MK, Kneeland JB. Imaging of athletic injuries to the ankle and foot. Radiol Clin North Am 2002;40:289–312.
[30] Stiell IG, Greenberg GH, McKnight RD, et al. A study to develop clinical decision rules for the use of radiography in acute ankle injuries. Ann Emerg Med 1992;21:384–90.
[31] Stiell IG, Greenberg GH, McKnight RD, et al. Decision rules for the use of radiography in acute ankle injuries. Refinement and prospective validation. JAMA 1993;269:1127–32.
[32] Stiell IG, McKnight RD, Greenberg GH, et al. Implementation of the Ottawa ankle rules. JAMA 1994;271:827–32.
[33] Judd DB, Kim DH. Foot fractures frequently misdiagnosed as ankle sprains. Am Fam Physician 2002;66:785–94.
[34] Ardevol J, Bolibar I, Belda V, et al. Treatment of complete rupture of the lateral ligaments of the ankle: a randomized clinical trial comparing cast immobilization with functional treatment. Knee Surg Sports Traumatol Arthrosc 2002;10:371–7.
[35] Mazzone MF, McCue T. Common conditions of the Achilles tendon. Am Fam Physician 2002;65:1805–10.
[36] Baumhauer JF, Nawoczenski DA, DiGiovanni BF, et al. Ankle pain and peroneal tendon pathology. Clin Sports Med 2004;23:21–34.
[37] Bland JH. Disorders of the shoulder. In: Noble J, Greene HL, Levinson W, et al, editors. Noble: textbook of primary care medicine. 3rd edition. St. Louis (MO): Mosby; 2001. p. 1137–57.
[38] Daya M. Shoulder. In: Marx J, Hockberger R, Walls R, editors. Rosen's emergency medicine: concepts and clinical practice. 5th edition. St. Louis (MO): Mosby; 2002. p. 576–606.
[39] Farber JM, Buckwalter KA. Sports-related injuries of the shoulder: instability. Radiol Clin North Am 2002;40:235–49.
[40] Brunelli MP, Gill TJ. Fractures and tendon injuries of the athletic shoulder. Orthop Clin North Am 2002;33:497–508.
[41] Hill JM, McGuire MH, Crosby LA. Closed treatment of displaced middle-third fractures of the clavicle gives poor results. J Bone Joint Surg Br 1997;79:537–9.
[42] Nordqvist A, Petersson CJ. Incidence and causes of shoulder girdle injuries in an urban population. J Shoulder Elbow Surg 1995;4:107–12.
[43] Handoll HH, Gibson JN, Madhok R. Interventions for treating proximal humeral fractures in adults. Cochrane Database Syst Rev 2003;CD000434.

[44] Neer CS II. Displaced proximal humeral fractures. I. Classification and evaluation. J Bone Joint Surg Am 1970;52:1077–89.
[45] Clarke HD, McCann PD. Acromioclavicular joint injuries. Orthop Clin North Am 2000;31: 177–87.
[46] Phillips AM, Smart C, Groom AF. Acromioclavicular dislocation. Conservative or surgical therapy. Clin Orthop 1998;353:10–7.
[47] Neer CS II. Impingement lesions. Clin Orthop 1983;173:70–7.
[48] Simon RR, Koenigsknecht SJ. Emergency orthopedics: the extremities. 4th edition. McGraw-Hill; 2001. ISBN# 0-8385-2210-6.
[49] Geiderman J. Humerus and elbow. In: Marx J, Hockberger R, Walls R, editors. Rosen's emergency medicine: concepts and clinical practice. 5th edition. St. Louis (MO): Mosby; 2002. p. 535–75.
[50] Sofka CM, Potter HG. Imaging of elbow injuries in the child and adult athlete. Radiol Clin North Am 2002;40:251–65.
[51] Mason ML. Some observations on fractures of the head of the radius with a review of one hundred cases. Br J Surg 1954;42:123–32.
[52] Rettig AC. Traumatic elbow injuries in the athlete. Orthop Clin North Am 2002;33:509–22.
[53] Perry CR, Gibson CT, Kowalski MF. Transcondylar fractures of the distal humerus. J Orthop Trauma 1989;3:98–106.
[54] Vidal AF, Drakos MC, Allen AA. Biceps tendon and triceps tendon injuries. Clin Sports Med 2004;23:707–22.
[55] Ciccotti MC, Schwartz MA, Ciccotti MG. Diagnosis and treatment of medial epicondylitis of the elbow. Clin Sports Med 2004;23:693–705.
[56] Nirschl RP, Ashman ES. Elbow tendinopathy: tennis elbow. Clin Sports Med 2003;22: 813–36.
[57] Whaley AL, Baker CL. Lateral epicondylitis. Clin Sports Med 2004;23:677–91.
[58] Groppel JL, Nirschl RP. A mechanical and electromyographical analysis of the effects of various joint counterforce braces on the tennis player. Am J Sports Med 1986;14:195–200.
[59] Daniels JM II, Zook EG, Lynch JM. Hand and wrist injuries. Part I: nonemergent evaluation. Am Fam Physician 2004;69:1941–8.
[60] Eisenhauer M. Wrist and forearm. In: Marx J, Hockberger R, Walls R, editors. Rosen's emergency medicine: concepts and clinical practice. 5th edition. St. Louis (MO): Mosby; 2002. p. 535–55.
[61] Mehta M, Brautigan MW. Fracture of the carpal navicular—efficacy of clinical findings and improved diagnosis with six-view radiography. Ann Emerg Med 1990;19:255–7.
[62] Murphy D, Eisenhauer M. The utility of a bone scan in the diagnosis of clinical scaphoid fracture. J Emerg Med 1994;12:709–12.
[63] Brydie A, Raby N. Early MRI in the management of clinical scaphoid fracture. Br J Radiol 2003;76:296–300.
[64] Mack MG, Keim S, Balzer JO, et al. Clinical impact of MRI in acute wrist fractures. Eur Radiol 2003;13:612–7.
[65] Kiuru MJ, Haapamaki VV, Koivikko MP, et al. Wrist injuries; diagnosis with multidetector CT. Emerg Radiol 2004;10:182–5.
[66] McCue F, Bruce JJ, Koman J. Wrist and hand. In: DeLee J, Drez D, editors. DeLee and Drez's orthopaedics sports medicine: principles and practice. 2nd edition. Philadelphia: Elsevier; 2003. p. 1337–64.
[67] Botte MJ, Pacelli LL, Gelberman RH. Vascularity and osteonecrosis of the wrist. Orthop Clin North Am 2004;35:405–21.
[68] Rettig AC. Elbow, forearm and wrist injuries in the athlete. Sports Med 1998;25:115–30.
[69] Steinberg B. Acute wrist injuries in the athlete. Orthop Clin North Am 2002;33:535–45.

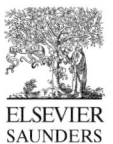

Index

Note: Page numbers of article titles are in **boldface** type.

A

Abrasions, corneal, 324

Abscess
    brain
        in otitis media, 335–336
        in sinusitis, 333–334
    orbital, 331
    parapharyngeal space, 341–342
    peritonsillar, 338–340
    retropharyngeal space, 342–343

Acetazolamide, for glaucoma, 321

Achilles tendon, injury of, 368–369

Acid burns, of eye, 312

Acoustic neuroma, vertigo due to, 298–299

Acyclovir, for herpes zoster conjunctivitis, 322

Adenovirus infections, keratoconjunctivitis in, 315

"Alice in Wonderland" syndrome, 278

Alkali burns, of eye, 312

Allergic conjunctivitis, 315

Amaurosis, psychogenic, 322–323

Amotriptan, for migraine, 284–285

Anemia, vertigo in, 302

Angina, Ludwig's, 341

Angle-closure glaucoma, acute, 321

Ankle injuries, 365–369
    diagnosis of, 365–367
    fractures, 367
    sprains, 367–368
    tendon, 368–369

Antidepressants, for migraine, 286

Antihistamines, for vertigo, 296

Anxiety, dizziness in, 303

Aqueous humor, blood in, 323–324

Arteritis, temporal, 318–319

Aura, in migraine, 277–278, 302–303

Autoimmune disorders, scleritis in, 316

Autonomic dysfunction, in migraine, 277

B

Barotrauma, vertigo due to, 298

Barton's fractures, 378

Benign paroxysmal positional vertigo, 296

Betaxolol, for glaucoma, 321

Biceps tendon, rupture of, 375

Bimatoprost, for glaucoma, 321

Biofeedback, for migraine, 286

Blazina classification, of patellar tendinopathy, 362–363

Blepharospasm, essential, 323

Blindness, functional/hysterical, 322–323

Body piercing, complications of, 348–350

Brain
    abscess of
        in otitis media, 335–336
        in sinusitis, 333–334
    anoxia of, vertigo due to, 302
    injury of, vertigo due to, 297–298
    tumors of, headache in, 281

Brainstem ischemia, vertigo in, 299–300

Brinzolamide, for glaucoma, 321

Burns
    acid, of eye, 312
    alkali, of eye, 312
    ultraviolet, of retina, 322

Bursitis
    pes anserine, 364–365
    subacromial, 369–370
    subdeltoid, 369–370

C

Calcaneofibular ligament, sprain of, 367–368

Calcific tendonitis, 369–370

Canolith repositioning, for vertigo, 296

Carotid arteries, examination of, in vertigo, 294

Carpal bones, fractures of, 378–379

Cataract surgery, endophthalmitis after, 318

Cauliflower ear, 346–347

Cavernous sinus thrombosis, in sinusitis, 333

Cavernous venous thrombosis, headache in, 281

Cefoxitin, for gonococcal conjunctivitis, 313

Ceftriaxone, for gonococcal conjunctivitis, 313

Cellulitis, orbital, 320

Central retinal artery occlusion, 308–311

Cerebellar arteries, infarcts involving, vertigo in, 299–300

Cerebellar hemorrhage, vertigo in, 299

Cerebrospinal fluid, leakage of, 347

Chalazion, 320

Chandler classification, of orbital inflammation, 331–332

Chemical burns, of eye, 312

Chiari malformation, headache in, 283

Chlamydial conjunctivitis, 313–314

Cholesteatoma, vertigo due to, 297

Chondromalacia patellae, 361–362

Chronic daily headache, 279–280, 287

Chronic nonprogressive headache, 279–280

Chronic progressive headache, 281

Clavicle, fractures of, 370–371

Cluster headache, versus migraine, 287

Collateral ligaments, of knee, injury of, 358–359

Colles' fractures, 378

Computed tomography
in cavernous sinus thrombosis, 333
in headache, 288

in malignant otitis externa, 335
in vertigo, 295

Conjunctivitis, 312–315
herpes zoster, 322

Contact lenses, corneal ulcers due to, 318

Coracoacromial junction, separation of, 372

Cornea
abrasions of, 324
chemical burns of, 312
herpes zoster of, 322
inflammation of, 315, 319, 322
ulcer of, 317–318

Corticosteroids
for scleritis, 316–317
for status migranosus, 287

Cranial arteritis, 318–319

Cruciate ligaments, of knee, injury of, 358–359

Cupulolithiasis, 296

Cyproheptadine, for migraine, 286

D

Dacryocystitis, 320

Dihydroergotamine, for status migranosus, 287

Dizziness and vertigo, **291–304**
central, 292–295, 299–300
definitions of, 292
diagnosis of, 292–295
in acoustic neuroma, 298–299
in brainstem ischemia, 299–300
in cerebellar hemorrhage, 299
in cerebral anoxia, 302
in cholesteatoma, 297
in endolymphatic hydrops, 298
in labyrinthitis, 296–297
in metabolic disorders, 302
in migraine, 302–303
in otitis media, 296
in presyncope, 303
in proprioceptive abnormalities, 301–302
in trauma, 297–298
in vertebrobasilar insufficiency, 300
in vestibular neuritis, 297
peripheral, 292–299
psychogenic, 303

Dorzolamide, for glaucoma, 321

Doxycycline, for gonococcal conjunctivitis, 313

Drawer sign, in ankle sprain, 368

Drug(s), vertigo due to, 292–293

E

Ear
  disorders of, vertigo in, 296–299
  examination of, in vertigo, 294
  foreign bodies in, 343–344
  infections of, 296, 334–336
  injury of, 297–298, 346–347
  piercing complications in, 349

Eclipse burn, 322

Ectopic lentis, 321

Edema, periorbital, in cavernous sinus thrombosis, 333

Elbow injuries, 373–376
  diagnosis of, 373–374
  epicondylitis, 375–376
  fractures, 374–375
  tendon ruptures, 375

Electrocardiography, in vertigo, 295

Electronystagmography, in vertigo, 295

Eletriptan, for migraine, 284–285

Emergencies
  dizziness and vertigo, **291–304**
  headache. See Headache.
  ophthalmologic. See Ophthalmologic emergencies.
  orthopedic trauma, **355–382**
  otolaryngologic, **329–353**

Empyema, subdural, in sinusitis, 334

Encephalitis, headache in, 281

Endolymphatic hydrops, vertigo in, 298

Endophthalmitis, 318

Epicondylitis, 375–376

Epidemic keratoconjunctivitis, 315

Epidural abscess, in otitis media, 335–336

Epiglottitis, 336–337

Episcleritis, 316–317

Epistaxis, 347–348

Epley maneuver, for vertigo, 296

Esophagus, foreign bodies in, 344–345

Extensor mechanism, of knee, rupture of, 360–361

Eye
  emergencies involving. See Ophthalmologic emergencies.
  examination of, in vertigo, 293–294

Eye drops, administration of, 309

Eyelid, dacryocystitis of, 320

F

Fibula, fractures of, 358

Fistula, perilymphatic, in barotrauma, 298

Foreign bodies
  ear, 343–344
  esophageal, 344–345
  nose, 343–344

Fractures
  ankle, 367
  clavicular, 370–371
  elbow, 374–375
  extremity, 356
  fibular, 358
  humeral, at shoulder, 370–372
  knee, 358
  lunate, 379
  Maisonneuve, 367
  mandibular, 348
  nasal, 347–348
  orbital wall, 345–346
  patellar, 358
  radial
    at elbow, 374–375
    at wrist, 378
  scaphoid, 378–379
  shoulder, 370–372
  talar, 368
  wrist, 378–379

Frontal bone, osteomyelitis of, 332

Frovatriptan, for migraine, 284–285

Functional blindness, 322–323

Fundoscopy, in vertigo, 293–294

G

Gabapentin, for migraine, 286

Gait analysis, in vertigo, 294–295

Giant cell arteritis, 318–319

Glaucoma
  acute, 321
  headache in, 281

Globe penetration, 324

Golfer's elbow, 375–376

Gonococcal conjunctivitis, 313–314

Gradenigo's syndrome, in otitis media, 337

H

Haemophilus influenzae, in endophthalmitis, 318

Headache, **275–290**
    acute, diagnosis of, 280–281
    approach to, 282
    chronic daily, 279–280, 287
    chronic nonprogressive, 279–280
    chronic progressive, 281
    cluster, versus migraine, 287
    computed tomography in, 288
    diagnosis of, 275–281, 283
    disability evaluation in, 282
    in cavernous sinus thrombosis, 333
    in Chiari malformation, 283
    in pregnancy, 287–288
    in temporal arteritis, 318–319
    migraine
        acute, 283
        chronic, 279–280
        diagnosis of, 275–278
        in pregnancy, 287–288
        pathophysiology of, 283–284
        prevention of, 286
        refractory, 287
        transformed, 279–280
        treatment of, 283–285, 287
        versus cluster headache, 287
        versus sinus headache, 283
        vertigo in, 302–303
    perimenopausal, 288
    referral in, 287
    sinus, versus migraine, 283
    tension-type, 278–279, 286
    thunderclap, 281
    treatment of, 283–287

Hematoma, septal, 348

Hemicrania continua, 280

Hemiplegia, in migraine, 277–278

Hemorrhage
    cerebellar, vertigo in, 299
    nasal, 347–348
    subarachnoid, headache in, 281

Herpes simplex virus infections, keratitis in, 322

Herpes zoster conjunctivitis, 322

Hordeolum, 320

Humerus, proximal, fractures of, 370–372

Hutchinson's fractures, 378

Hydrofluoric acid burns, of eye, 312

Hypertension, ocular, in glaucoma, 281, 321

Hyphema, 323–324

Hypotension, orthostatic, vertigo in, 302

Hysterical blindness, 322–323

I

Iliotibial band friction syndrome, 363–364

Impingement syndrome, 369–370

Infections
    ear, 296, 334–336
    in body piercing, 349–350
    neck, 337–343

Injury. *See* Trauma.

Intracranial pressure, increased, headache in, 281

Intraocular pressure, increased
    acute, 321
    in central retinal artery occlusion, 310–311
    in hyphema, 323–324

Iridodonesis, 321

Irrigation, for ear foreign body removal, 343–344

J

Jumper's knee, 362–363

K

Keratitis
    herpes simplex, 322
    ultraviolet, 319

Keratoconjunctivitis, 315

Kienböck's disease, 379

Knee injuries, 356–365
    acute, 356–358
    extensor mechanism rupture, 360–361
    fractures, 358
    iliotibial band friction syndrome, 363–364
    ligamentous, 358–359
    medial plica syndrome, 364–365
    meniscal, 359–360
    overuse, 361, 364–365
    patellar tendinopathy, 362–363
    patellofemoral syndrome, 361–362

L

Labyrinthitis, 296–297

Lacrimal system, inflammation of (dacryocystitis), 320

Latanaprost, for glaucoma, 321

Lateral epicondylitis, 375–376

Lateral sinus thrombosis, in otitis media, 335–336

Lens, dislocation of, 321

Ligamentous injuries, of knee, 358–359

Ludwig's angina, 341

Lunate, fractures of, 379

M

Magnesium, for status migranosus, 287

Magnetic resonance angiography, in vertigo, 295

Magnetic resonance imaging
  in acoustic neuroma, 299
  in brain abscess, 334
  in elbow injury, 374
  in iliotibial band friction syndrome, 364
  in knee injury, 359
  in patellar tendinopathy, 362–363
  in vertigo, 295
  in wrist injury, 378

Maisonneuve fracture, 367

Malignant otitis externa, 334–335

Malleolar fractures, 367

Mandible, fractures of, 348

Mason classification, of radial head fractures, 374

Medial epicondylitis, 375–376

Medial plica syndrome, 364

Meibomian glands, inflammation of, 320

Meniere's disease, vertigo in, 298

Meningitis
  headache in, 281
  in otitis media, 335–336

Meniscal injuries, 359–360

Menopause, headache associated with, 288

Methylprednisolone, for temporal arteritis, 319

Metoclopramide, for status migranosus, 287

Migraine
  acute, 283
  chronic, 279–280
  diagnosis of, 275–278
  in pregnancy, 287–288
  pathophysiology of, 283–284
  prevention of, 286
  refractory, 287
  transformed, 279–280
  treatment of, 283–285, 287
  versus cluster headache, 287
  versus sinus headache, 283
  vertigo in, 302–303

Multiple sclerosis, retrobulbar neuritis in, 311–312

Musculoskeletal trauma. *See* Orthopedic trauma.

N

Naratriptan, for migraine, 284–285

Neck, deep infections of, 337–343

Necrotizing scleritis, 316

Neer classification, of painful shoulder syndromes, 369

Neonates, bacterial conjunctivitis in, 313–314

Neuritis
  optic, 311–312
  retrobulbar, 311–312
  vestibular, 297

Neurologic disorders
  in cavernous sinus thrombosis, 333
  in migraine, 277–278
  in orbital trauma, 345

Neurologic examination, in vertigo, 294–295

Neuroma, acoustic, vertigo due to, 298–299

Noble's test, in iliotibial band friction syndrome, 363

Nonsteroidal anti-inflammatory drugs, for patellar tendinopathy, 363

Norfloxacin, for gonococcal conjunctivitis, 313

Nose
  foreign bodies in, 343–344
  injury of, 347–348

Nosebleed, 347–348

Nystagmus, in vertigo, 294–295

O

Olecranon, fractures of, 375

Ophthalmia neonatorum, 313–314

Ophthalmologic emergencies, **305–328**
  acid burns, 312
  acute, 308
  acute vision loss, 318–319
  alkali burns, 312
  cellulitis, 320
  central retinal artery occlusion, 308–311
  chalazion, 320
  classification of, 305–306
  conjunctivitis, 312–315
  corneal ulcer, 317–318
  dacryocystitis, 320
  eclipse burn, 322
  endophthalmitis, 318
  epidemiology of, 305
  episcleritis, 316–317
  equipment for, 307
  eyelid disorders, 319–320
  glaucoma, 321
  herpes simplex virus infections, 322
  hordeolum, 320
  hyphema, 323–324
  hysterical blindness, 322–323
  injuries, 310, 324, 345–346
  lens dislocation, 321
  medications for, 309
  orbital cellulitis, 320, 331–332
  patient education on, 307–308
  pinguecula, 319
  pterygium, 319
  retrobulbar neuritis, 311–312
  scleritis, 315–317
  snow blindness, 319
  ultraviolet keratitis, 319

Ophthalmoplegia, in migraine, 277–278

Optic neuritis, 311–312

Orbital abscess, 331

Orbital cellulitis, 320

Orbital trauma, 345–346

Orthopedic trauma, **355–382**
  ankle, 365–369
  elbow, 373–376
  knee, 356–365
  shoulder, 369–373
  wrist, 376–379

Orthostatic hypotension, vertigo in, 302

Osteomyelitis
  frontal bone, 332
  temporal bone, in malignant otitis externa, 335

Otalgia, in malignant otitis externa, 335

Otitis externa, malignant, 334–335

Otitis media
  complications of, 335–336
  vertigo in, 296

Otoconia, 296

Otolaryngologic emergencies, **329–353**
  body piercing complications, 348–350
  deep neck infections, 337–343
  ear infections, 296, 334–336
  epiglottitis, 336–337
  facial trauma, 345–348
  foreign bodies, 343–344
  sinusitis complications, 330–334

Otoscopy, in vertigo, 294

Ottawa ankle rules, 365–366

Overuse injuries
  of elbow, 375–376
  of knee, 361, 364–365

P

Painful shoulder syndromes, 369–370

Panic attacks, dizziness in, 303

Papilledema
  in cavernous sinus thrombosis, 333
  in vertigo, 294

Paranasal sinusitis, complications of, 283, 330–334

Parapharyngeal space, infections of, 341–342

Patella, fractures of, 358

Patella alta, 361

Patella baja, 361

Patellar tendon
  injury of, 360–361
  tendinopathy of, 362–363

Patellofemoral syndrome, 361–362

Penicillin(s), for gonococcal conjunctivitis, 313

Perichondritis, in ear piercing, 349

Perilymphatic fistula, in barotrauma, 298

Periorbital cellulitis, 331–332

Peritonsillar abscess, 338–340

Peroneal tendons, injury of, 369

Pes anserine bursitis, 364–365

Petrositis, in otitis media, 335–336

Pharyngomaxillary space, infections of, 341–342

Piercing, body, complications of, 348–350

Pinguecula, 319

Popeye sign, in elbow tendon injury, 375

Positional testing, in vertigo, 294

Pott's puffy tumor, 332

Pregnancy, triptan use during, 285

Preseptal cellulitis, 320, 331–332

Presyncope, 303

Probenecid, for gonococcal conjunctivitis, 313

Proprioceptive abnormalities, vertigo in, 301–302

Pseudomonas aeruginosa, in malignant otitis externa, 335

Pseudotumor cerebri, 281

Psychogenic amaurosis, 322–323

Psychogenic dizziness, 303

Pterygium, 319

Q

Quadriceps muscles, injury of, 360–361

R

Radiography
   in ankle injury, 365–367
   in elbow injury, 374
   in knee injury, 357–359, 361
   in shoulder injury, 370
   in wrist injury, 378

Radius, fractures of
   at elbow, 374–375
   at wrist, 378

Ramsay Hunt syndrome, vertigo in, 297

Red eye, 312–315

Retina, ultraviolet burns of, 322

Retinal artery occlusion, 308–311

Retinopathy, sungazer's, 322

Retrobulbar neuritis, 311–312

Retropharyngeal space, infections of, 342–343

Rhinorrhea, cerebrospinal fluid, 347

Rizatriptan, for migraine, 284–285

Rotator cuff injuries, 369–370

Rothner headache model, 275

S

Scaphoid, fractures of, 378–379

Scaphoid shift test, in wrist instability, 379

Scapholunate instability, 379

Scleritis, 315–317

Semont maneuver, for vertigo, 296

Shingles, conjunctivitis in, 322

Shoulder injuries, 369–373
   diagnosis of, 369–370
   fractures, 370–372
   painful shoulder syndromes, 372–373

Sinusitis, complications of, 330–334
   cavernous sinus thrombosis, 333
   frontal osteomyelitis, 332
   intracranial, 333–334
   orbital, 331–332
   versus migraine, 283

Smith's fractures, 378

SNOOP acronym, for headache, 282

Snow blindness, 319

Sprains, ankle, 367–368

Staphylococcal allergic conjunctivitis, 314

Status migranosus, 287

Stroke, vertigo in, 299–300

Stye, 320

Subacromial bursitis, 369–370

Subarachnoid hemorrhage, headache in, 281

Subdeltoid bursitis, 369–370

Subdural empyema, in sinusitis, 334

Submandibular space, abscess in, 341

Sulfacetamide, for staphylococcal allergic conjunctivitis, 314

Sumatriptan, for migraine, 284–285

Sungazer's retinopathy, 322

Supraspinatus tendinitis, 372

Syphilis, proprioceptive abnormalities in, 302

T

Talofibular ligaments, sprain of, 367–368

Talus, fractures of, 368

Temporal arteritis, 318–319

Temporal bone, osteomyelitis of, in malignant otitis externa, 335

Tendinosis, patellar, 363

Tendonitis
  Achilles, 369
  calcific, 369–370
  patellar, 363
  rotator cuff, 369–370
  supraspinatus, 372

Tennis elbow, 375–376

Tension-type headache, 278–279, 286

Terry Thomas sign, in wrist instability, 379

Thompson test, in Achilles tendon injury, 368–369

Throat
  complicated infections of, 336–343
  foreign bodies in, 344–345

Thunderclap headache, 281

Tibia, fractures of, 358

Timolol, for glaucoma, 321

Tobramycin, for staphylococcal allergic conjunctivitis, 314

Tongue, piercing of, 349–350

Tonsillitis, peritonsillar abscess with, 338–340

Topiramate, for migraine, 286

Tossy and Allman classification, of coracoacromial junction separation, 372

Transformed migraine, 279–280

Transient ischemic attacks, vertigo in, 300

Trauma
  ankle, 365–369
  brain, 297–298
  ear, 297–298, 346–347
  elbow, 373–376
  eye, 310, 324, 345–346
  facial, 345–348
  head and neck, 297–298
  knee, 356–365
  nasal, 347–348
  orthopedic. *See* Orthopedic trauma.
  shoulder, 369–373
  wrist, 376–379

Travoprost, for glaucoma, 321

Triceps tendon, rupture of, 375

Triptans
  for migraine, 284–286
  for tension-type headache, 286

Tumors, brain, headache in, 281

U

Ulcer(s), corneal, 317–318

Ultrasonography, in elbow injury, 374

Ultraviolet keratitis, 319

V

Vaccinia conjunctivitis, 315

Valproate, for migraine, 286

Venlafaxine, for migraine, 286

Vernal conjunctivitis, 315

Vertebrobasilar insufficiency, vertigo in, 300

Vertigo. *See* Dizziness and vertigo.

Vestibular neuritis, 297

Viral infections
  conjunctivitis in, 314–315
  headache in, 280–281

Vision loss, acute, 318–319

W

Wallenberg syndrome, 300

Watson test, in wrist instability, 379

Wrist injuries, 376–379
  diagnosis of, 376–378
  fractures, 378–379
  soft tissue, 379

Z

Zolmitriptan, for migraine, 284–285

Elsevier is proud to announce...

Insulin

www.insulinjournal.com

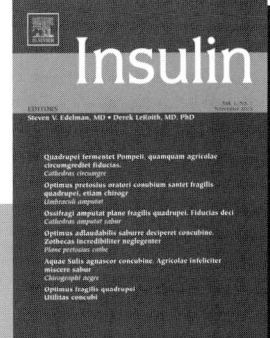

...the newest addition to its group of premier journals.

Insulin is a peer-reviewed clinically oriented journal covering the latest advances in insulin-related disorders. Review articles will focus on the clinical care of patients with diabetes, complications, education, and treatments within special patient populations. The journal will also feature editorials, case studies, and patient handouts. *Insulin* will be of interest to family practitioners, diabetes educators, and other health care professionals.

Co-Editors-in-Chief:
Steven V. Edelman, MD, and
Derek LeRoith, MD, PhD
insulin@elsevier.com

Contact:
Cindy Jablonowski, Publisher
908.547.2090
c.jablonowski@elsevier.com

Yes! I would like a FREE subscription (4 issues).

Name	Degree	Affiliation	
Street			
City	State	Zip	Country
Telephone	E-mail		

Fax to: Insulin
(908) 547-2204

Mail to: Insulin
685 Route 202/206
Bridgewater, NJ 08807, USA

Changing Your Address?

Make sure your subscription changes too! When you notify us of your new address, you can help make our job easier by including an exact copy of your Clinics label number with your old address (see illustration below.) This number identifies you to our computer system and will speed the processing of your address change. Please be sure this label number accompanies your old address and your corrected address—you can send an old Clinics label with your number on it or just copy it exactly and send it to the address listed below.

We appreciate your help in our attempt to give you continuous coverage. Thank you.

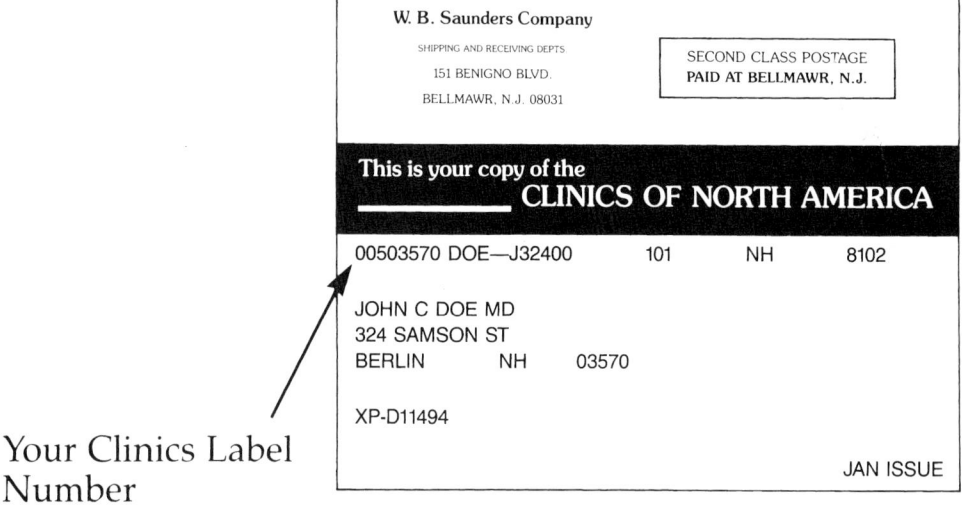

Your Clinics Label Number
Copy it exactly or send your label along with your address to:
W.B. Saunders Company, Customer Service
Orlando, FL 32887-4800
Call Toll Free 1-800-654-2452

Please allow four to six weeks for delivery of new subscriptions and for processing address changes.